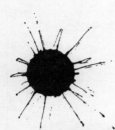

CAUGHT SHORT

CAUGHT SHORT

When nature calls & you've nowhere to hide

Dan Crompton

First published in Great Britain in 2013 by
Michael O'Mara Books Limited
9 Lion Yard
Tremadoc Road
London SW4 7NQ

Copyright © Dan Crompton 2013

A CIP catalogue record for this book is available from
the British Library.

Papers used by Michael O'Mara Books Limited are
natural, recyclable products made from wood grown
in sustainable forests. The manufacturing processes
conform to the environmental regulations of the
country of origin.

ISBN: 978-1-78243-045-2 in paperback print format

1 2 3 4 5 6 7 8 9 10

www.mombooks.com

Designed and typeset by Blok Graphic

Printed and bound by CPI Group (UK) Ltd,
Croydon, CR0 4YY

Contents

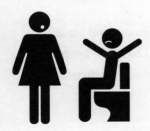

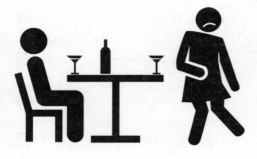

Introduction

Everyone has that one embarrassing story that's always reeled out through wine-stained lips at the end of a dinner party, or during a particularly traumatic game of Truth or Dare. It's generally prefixed with, 'I've never told anybody this, but . . .' and followed by an outpouring of even worse stories from the rest of the assembled company.

Having attended far too many boozy dinners, and having played far too many games of Truth or Dare with people I shouldn't have, I am able to collate the most horrendous and appalling stories I have been told.

Many thanks to everyone who has been brave or drunk enough to share their appalling stories with me – and sincere apologies to those whose names I couldn't be bothered to change . . .

There are even a couple of my own personal horrors among these pages, but I can assure you that they have been penned under a pseudonym.

Hear more stories or share your own horrors online . . .

 /CaughtShort

 #Caught_Short

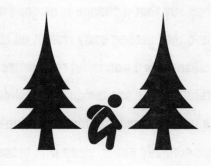

PART ONE:
Travelling Nightmares

They say that a change is as good as a rest, and that getting away from it all to sunnier climes has a wonderful restorative effect. Unfortunately, the excitement of a holiday tends to give us a renewed confidence to drink more than we normally would, sleep with greasy and unattractive bar staff (just me?), and eat food from street vendors that we wouldn't otherwise touch with a bargepole (just where do they wash their hands when they've gone for a piss?).

The upshot of this, however, is a wealth of wonderful woes that will have you burning your passport in no time.

Vindaloo

BEN M.

A mate and I were travelling through India last year, and were on a long train journey heading out of Mumbai. We'd both got a bit of the 'Delhi Belly', but I was suffering worse by far. The train was rammed full of people, and I suddenly had the imminent urge to go to the toilet – and it wasn't going to wait.

It took an age for us to climb through all the people along two carriages, and when we finally reached the loo, I found it was busy. I started pumping sweat. Suddenly this was an emergency. In my blind panic, the only thing I could think of was to lower a window and ask my mate to lift me up so I could get my arse outside of the train.

The relief as I shat down the outside of the carriage was unbelievable – but was immediately replaced with complete horror as I realized the train was slowing down and pulling alongside a packed platform.

If the story ended there it'd be bad enough, but sadly no. I was laughing so hard that I lost what little control I still had over my bodily functions and pissed all over my mate, who was still holding me up.

Sock story #1

MARK

I was in the middle of nowhere in Ireland for a wedding a few years back, and was driving myself back to the airport. Soon after I'd set off, my enjoyment of the stunning landscape was hampered somewhat by a distinct suspicion that I should have gone to the bathroom while I was still near civilization.

There weren't any roadside restaurants and the only sign of life at the one petrol station I passed was a couple of sheep grazing on the forecourt, and the next sign to the airport showed I still had a good hour in the car – so I figured there was only one thing for it.

It was pissing down, but I stopped the car beside a large bush and ran behind it to answer nature's call. My immense relief was short-lived when I realized I didn't have anything to wipe myself with except twigs and leaves – which for reasons I still can't fathom seemed a less attractive option than using one of my own socks. And then the other one, too.

To this day I can't quite work out what the fuck I was thinking in using the socks, but I know I will never understand what I hoped to achieve by then shoving the soggy, shitty things into my sports bag. But anyway, I was late for my plane so I drove on and basically forgot all about it.

Not for long, alas, because when I finally made it to the departure gate, soaked to the skin and sweating profusely, the security guy pulled me over and said, 'I'm going to have to check your bag, sir.'

As he started yanking the zip, it seemed only polite to tell him, 'Good luck!'

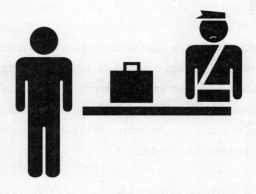

The water park

KATH

My brother got married last summer. I knew his fiancée reasonably well, but not well enough to socialize with independently of my brother. Under the obligation of some unwritten rule, she was kind enough to invite me to her hen party holiday in Spain. And through the same obligation, I was duty-bound to attend.

The maid of honour and other bridesmaids had gone to quite some effort to ensure that no moment of the long weekend went unfilled – and so I found myself on a relentless sequence of shots, drinking games and penis-shaped apparatus with a bunch of girls three years my junior.

I compensated for being somewhat an outsider by getting fully stuck in with the drinking on the first night – something I regretted severely the next morning, when our rigid schedule forced us into an early start for the day's planned activities.

We all descended upon an out-of-town water park for the day. And with one of the worst hangovers of my life, it was my idea of hell in a bikini. After a particularly greasy lunch, we climbed up to one of the park's many water flumes.

I was the first one down the slide. The overwhelming combination of the lunch mixed with rolling around down the twists of that flume was all too much. I lost all control of my body and was spectacularly sick down the inside of the slide as I continued to swish down.

I turned around just in time to see the remaining girls come whizzing round the corner in a chain, and the split-second horror on their faces as they slid straight through the trail of puke behind me.

Shakes on a plane

EMMA P.

A couple of years ago, my boyfriend and I were flying home from our first holiday together in Dubai. Despite my fears of any awkwardness, the holiday had gone really well so far.

The flight was long, and we hit a bit of turbulence over Europe. Our seats were towards the front of the plane, so when the turbulence settled down a bit, I walked shakily up the aisle and into the first available loo.

My boyfriend had been dozing off, so I thought I would get away with a number two.

As I sat in the tiny cubicle, the plane started shaking again, and the pilot made the announcement for all passengers to return to their seats. Unfortunately, I was very much in the middle of something, and had no choice but to finish the job.

Just as I leant forwards to wipe my bum, the plane lurched suddenly down and to the side, and I was at once launched forwards into the door – which turned out not to be properly locked – and onto the floor outside with my skirt and knickers round my ankles. Oh God!

Mortified, I instantly tried to get up, but a final lurch of the plane sent me rolling down the aisle up to the first row of seats, with my unwiped arse on display. In a blind panic, I yanked my skirt up and ran back into the cubicle, with the image of 250 horrified faces looking down at me burnt into my eyes.

In one quick move, I wiped myself and sank down on the seat with my head in my hands. I absently reached behind me to activate the flush – and within seconds, the vacuum action had sucked me right down into the toilet, with my arse pressed against the cold, wet metal of the bowl. With another five hours left of the flight, I have never wanted a shower more in my life.

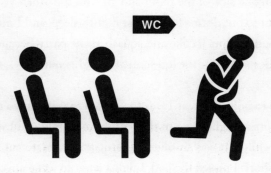

Summer damp

MICHELLE M.

I was a bit of a funny kid, and found it difficult to make friends at school, so I used to go to summer camps during the long school holidays. One year, when I was about fourteen years old, there was actually another girl from my school going. We weren't very good friends at all, but our mums got wind of it somehow and arranged that they would split the car journeys between them. So I made the journey to the camp in her mum's car, and we barely spoke the whole ride – nor for rest of the two-week camp.

I had a good time as usual, and the last night always culminated in one of those school-disco style parties, with boys on one side of the room and girls on the other. We later all went to our dorms for the last night's sleep, and I must have had too much coke and squash at the party, because I was desperate for the loo soon after lights out.

I tried to hold it out, as I was too scared to walk down the corridors at night to go to the bathroom. (I told you I was a funny child.) It was absolutely excruciating and, to cut a long story short: I pissed the bed. I didn't want to wake anyone up and embarrass myself, so took my dressing gown from the floor and lay on top of that for the rest of the night.

The following morning, I packed my suitcase and stuffed the damp dressing gown into my holdall. My mum eventually came to pick us up, and the two of us girls made our way over to the car to awkwardly sit in silence as my mum was busying herself getting our bags into the boot. Then I heard her ask from behind us, 'Why is your dressing gown so wet?' as she pulled it out of my holdall.

I was mortified, blushing, and hoped to God none of the other kids could see this. I made up some excuse about spilling some water on it this morning. My mother couldn't bear the thought of stuffing a wet dressing gown back into a bag for the three-hour drive, and so (despite my protestations) she tied it by the arms to the roof rack of our car for it to dry.

I spent the whole of the journey staring out of the car window, absolutely horrified at the fact that my piss-covered dressing gown was billowing in the wind above our heads all the way home.

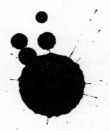

Greek dip

NICK

When I was in my early twenties I went on a lads' holiday
to Greece with a few mates. It had inevitably turned into an
unceasing cycle of drinking and trying to get laid – one more
than the other in my case. On our penultimate day, we had
booked ourselves on to a boozy boat trip on a catamaran –
one of those all-day boat trips to nowhere, with fifty pissed-
up Brits flirting, drinking and ultimately vomiting overboard.
This one was not to disappoint.

After an hour or so, the cocktails had certainly hit, and we
were standing under the canopy chatting up a group of
nice-enough-looking girls. With absolutely no warning
whatsoever, my stomach suddenly gave way, and I had quite
simply just shat myself. It must have been a combination

of dodgy food and a week of non-stop booze that caused the unannounced explosion.

I hoped I could get away with it; there were a lot of people there, with loud music, and the sea breeze carrying away most of the stench. But I could feel the wetness making its way down my legs, and about to creep out the bottom of my shorts. To compound the horror, my pants felt well and truly wet, and of course – of course! – I was wearing white fucking shorts.

I had two options of how to deal with the hideous situation: either to drop my drink and jump overboard in a spontaneous act of wackiness, or to find my way to the catamaran toilet and sort myself out. The former would certainly have been cleaner, but I couldn't guarantee I wouldn't be stranded at sea, nor that the entire boatload of people wouldn't see my browning shorts as I leapt overboard. So I made a swift excuse and waddled through the party to the tiny toilet cubicle below deck with my arse clenched, trying to style out the fact that I was covered in my own diarrhoea.

When I locked the door, I found that there was no fucking toilet paper in the cubicle. This was a nightmare. I had no choice but to vaguely clean my shitty pants under the slow trickle of the tap and use them to wipe down the insides of my shorts. I got them to a stage where they were certainly wet, definitely slightly brown, but not completely covered in shit. That would have to do. The next task was to dispose of the pants.

In my pissed mind, flushing them down the toilet was the best option. However, the pump-action flush of the catamaran toilet only made them slightly blue with disinfectant and they didn't budge. So the only option I had was to open the cistern behind the loo and hide them in there. Coming out, with wet and slightly brown shorts, I waddled back into the party and counted down the minutes before we got back on dry land.

A New York state

HELEN

I was nineteen and alone in New York on the second-to-last day of my gap year travels. I had been taken under the wing of some older guys in the hostel, thanks to whom I was now at a secret keg party and terribly, terribly drunk. My head was doing the bad kind of spinning – waves of hideousness rolling up and over. After an inevitable snog with the most hideous boy I've ever clapped eyes on, I decided it was time for bed.

Sadly the five Israeli guys with whom I was sharing my dorm had sensibly gone to sleep hours ago. I 'quietly' let myself into the pitch-black room and 'crept' towards my bunk, where I lay silently hiccupping and clutching my head in an attempt to stop everything from spinning.

Suddenly I knew I was going to be sick. I leapt up, crashed into the opposite bunk, tripped over something and fell headlong into the bathroom. I stuck my face into the loo and puked up about nineteen pints of beer, all the while sobbing in the usual ladylike manner. I was such a state by the end of this that I couldn't work out how to flush the loo or turn the taps on to wash my hands. I stumbled out into the dorm,

where the Israelis were doing a cracking job of pretending
to be asleep, and shook my bunkmate awake. We had never
so much as said hello and here I was breathing vomit fumes
in his face at 3 a.m. Chivalrously he went into the bathroom
and either did or didn't sort the mess out – I have no idea as
I fell into bed and passed out.

I woke up alone next morning – my last day before flying
home – to the most glorious blue-skied New York day.
It was awful. I shut the curtains and put my sunglasses
on. My mouth tasted like arse. I fumbled my way to the
bathroom to brush my teeth. No water. Neither tap would
produce anything and even the toilet cistern was empty.
Clearly the water had been cut off. I started sobbing again.

Eventually I managed to make it downstairs – good thing
I was still wearing my clothes and shoes from the night
before – and the receptionist confirmed that the whole block
had indeed had the water shut off. The hostel toilets were
out of bounds until further notice. I simply had to get some
water so I wobbled down the street to the nearest shop. The
British newspapers on sale there were covered in photos of
TV presenter Jill Dando, who'd been killed the previous day,
so I bought the *Mail* and some bottled water and life-giving
salty crisps and retired to my hostel's sunny roof terrace.

I was just starting to feel vaguely alive again when I was overwhelmed with the need to poo. But I wasn't allowed to use the bathrooms and there wasn't a McDonald's or Starbucks within dashing distance. This was turning into the worst day of my life. I realized I had no choice: I was going to have to make illegal use of the hostel's facilities. I grabbed my things and staggered inside to the nearest bathroom – fortunately for the long-suffering Israelis, I was a few flights up from my own room – only to discover that other people had clearly had the same idea. The toilet was practically overflowing and there was no paper left either.

But there was no time to waste. I sat down and got on with it – I'll spare the details but needless to say it was quite something – and then, muttering apologetic RIPs to the soul of poor Jill Dando, wiped my arse with her face.

Delhi Belly

BRADLEY S.

Anyone who has travelled to India will know the horror
of an unavoidable bout of Delhi Belly. No matter how
careful you are, it is an inevitable rite of passage for any
India newbie.

I was waiting on a busy station platform with my group
of friends, with our huge backpacks on our backs, waiting
for our long-distance train to pull in. I had not been well
for a day or so, although it had been fairly manageable
as long as I was within dashing distance of a toilet. But
it was getting slowly worse, until I had about a fifteen-
second warning between thinking, 'I could quite do with a
shit,' to it actually happening, whether I was ready or not.

In this instance, I was not.

The train was pulling in, and there was no way I could
make it to the station toilet in time. And I shat myself –
right there on the busy platform. It was largely contained,
but nonetheless wet, and I decided to style it out without
saying a word while we all shoved (or waddled) to get on
to the train.

Once on board, I made an immediate excuse to find the toilet cubicle a couple of carriages down, squelching through the travellers and families that filled the train. In the toilet, I made the best I could of the situation, removing my pants and wiping down the inside of my trousers. I had nowhere to hide the shitty underwear, so could only think to open the window and hurl them out as we hurtled through the city. I then counted down the hours before I could finally have a shower.

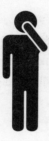

I had about a fifteen-second warning between thinking, 'I could quite do with a shit,' to it actually happening, whether I was ready or not.

Top o' the vommin'

JACK L.

There's not much preamble to this story: it was my cousin's eighteenth birthday, and also St Patrick's Day, so a bunch of us had flown from Manchester to Dublin for a night on the Guinness. We must have drunk at least ten pints by the time my cousin announced he was off for a puke and stumbled through the crowd to the gents. His brother and I thought it'd be a laugh to go and take the piss out of him, so we trooped off in hot pursuit.

We found him locked in the middle cubicle and there were suitably anguished noises coming from within, so we took up our positions on the toilet seats on either side and peered over the cubicle walls, cheering him on.

There's only so long you can maintain a keen interest in watching someone vomit, though, and his brother decided it was time to ramp things up a bit.

'Tell you what,' he said to me, 'if you eat a fingerful of his puke, I'll buy you a Guinness.'

Well, a pint's a pint, right?

Green Kwai curry

WARREN S.

My mate Joe and I had been travelling around Thailand for a month and were spending a few days in a cabin by the River Kwai. Late one night we'd had a couple of beers and smokes and were sitting by the water admiring the moon and the stars on the ripples and all that shite when I decided to dive in for a refreshing swim. It felt amazing and I couldn't believe how lucky I was to be there.

The next day my shit was green. It stayed that way for two weeks, and I was actually so incapacitated that we had to cancel the next few stages of our trip so that I could get medical attention. I couldn't even fart without following through. The look on the doctor's face when Joe told him

I'd been swimming in the Kwai was, in hindsight, priceless.
It turned out there was a massive sewage pipe spewing
its load into the river about twelve inches from where
I'd jumped in.

After a few weeks of extreme diarrhoea and dehydration,
I felt it was safe enough to resume normal service, so Joe and
I hired some motorbikes and took off for our first day out
in ages. It felt brilliant. So brilliant, in fact, that I thought
I'd celebrate by risking my first fart in weeks.

It was not a success.

I came to an emergency stop and whipped off my shitty
boxers at the side of the road. Joe was off his bike and pissing
himself – sadly not literally – but every time I laughed it
unleashed more shit. I wasn't even sure if I was laughing
or sobbing. I chucked my boxers in the storage area under
my motorbike seat and we carried on.

The next day we were finally going to be on our way
again, so we dropped the bikes off back at the rental place.
We were safely ensconced on our bus by the time I realized
I'd forgotten to retrieve my little package. Oops.

Brownwash

JAMIE T.

My girlfriend and I had recently arrived in India as part of a
round-the-world backpacking trip and had enthusiastically
thrown ourselves into all that the country had to offer –
including, in my case, a horrific dose of Delhi Belly. I have
never in my life felt so close to death's door. I was confined
to a dirty mattress in our windowless room for two days,
sweating and delirious, and only rousing myself every couple
of hours to stagger out to the communal bathroom. The
slightest attempt at nutrition – a sip of water, even – had
me doubled up with stomach cramps.

On the third day my girlfriend had gone off to look at
some temple or other on her own. I couldn't trust myself
in the outside world and assured her I'd be fine in my
darkened cave. About half an hour in, I must have inhaled
too much oxygen or something because my stomach
suddenly convulsed in pain. I climbed up off the mattress,
groaning and making old-man noises, and staggered out
of the room.

I got to the bathroom to find both cubicles taken. I was so
weak that I wanted to cry. I knew there was an Internet cafe

next to the hostel so I decided I'd just have to go there.
I staggered out, skinny and pale and blinded by the sun,
and was almost knocked back by the sounds and smells
of the street. It was all too much for my feeble stomach.
I ducked into a little alleyway between the hostel and the
cafe, pulled down my shorts and – forgive the detail –
sprayed shit all over the whitewashed wall. Tourists stopped
and watched in horror and I whimpered at them to go away.

My girlfriend returned later, full of tales of palaces and
monkeys and toothless old men, to find me in surprisingly
good spirits. I was on the mend at last.

The next day I led her to the scene of my disgrace and
proudly showed her where the paint on the previously
pristine wall had been corroded off by my shit. She dutifully
took a photo.

We hid that picture when we showed our parents the
holiday snaps, but strangely it was the only one my mates
wanted to see.

If I can make it there . . .

<u>HAZEL L.</u>

My brother and I were in our mid-twenties and had just arrived in New York for an exciting first visit when I started to feel horribly unwell. When I say we'd just arrived I mean we had literally just arrived: we were standing right at the back of an insanely long immigration queue waiting to have our fingers and eyeballs scanned. By the time I got to the stern-looking guy in the little kiosk I was pale and sweating and could barely keep my eyes open. For some reason he let me into the country, and I celebrated by shuffling to the nearest bathroom and emitting a great quantity of diarrhoea.

Much the same thing happened on the other side of baggage claim, and on the way to the taxi rank, and within seconds of getting to our hotel. I finally held it in long enough to find a pharmacy and dose myself up on Imodium, and off we went to the Empire State Building.

We'd made it about four blocks before I needed to find a toilet again. I dashed into a McDonald's. Two blocks later I undid the good work of the bathroom attendant at a

Starbucks. Finally, within sight of the Empire State Building – actually, our hotel was within sight of the Empire State Building, it had just taken us half an hour to get there – I ran wildly into a packed Burger King, clutching my stomach. Clearly they had seen me coming because the customer cubicle was securely locked. I begged one of the servers to open it for me, by this point in tears, and was eventually admitted into the only Manhattan attraction I cared about in that instant.

I was mid-shit, farting and groaning, when the door swung open and a man and his two kids started coming in. They were carrying balloons. They screamed. From my vantage point I could literally see the food being prepared behind them and happy customers, ready to enjoy their delicious meals, turning from the counter to see what the commotion was all about, then holding their hands to their noses. I heard one woman say, 'Oh my God, honey, what is that?' But there was nothing I could do to stop the torrent of horror, or indeed excrement.

'It wasn't supposed to be like thiiiiiiiiis!' I wailed deliriously, as New York slammed its door in my face.

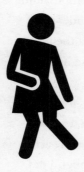

Urine luck

POPPY M.

During my gap year I spent a couple of weeks in Sydney, sharing a hostel room on Bondi Beach with eleven revolting but lovable British blokes. I knew they'd accepted me as one of their own when I left them partying in the room as I went to bed one night and then woke up at 3 a.m. because they were trying to drop a Mars Bar down the back of my PJs so that I'd think I'd shat myself.

Anyway, we were there during Sydney's annual Mardi Gras parade. The boys and I spent the afternoon drinking in the sunshine and then headed to Hyde Park in the evening and climbed a tree for a better view. This all seemed very hilarious at the time, especially when the police turned up twice to tell us we were contravening health and safety regulations, until we all realized we needed to pee. The lads all wandered off into the park and pissed wherever the fancy took them before cracking open another beer, but being a girl I had higher standards. Or so I insisted.

I clenched determinedly and marched off in the direction of one of the major thoroughfares, knowing I'd come across a Maccy D's or similar before too long. Sure enough I did, but evidently at least 9,000 other women had had the same thought; I pushed through the throng of jiggling, cross-legged women only to find the bathroom had been closed off. All the other potential, er, 'watering holes' along the street had signs on the front door saying the loos were out of bounds.

By now things were looking pretty desperate. I walk-ran back through the park – momentum seemed to stop the contents of my bladder from sloshing around too much – and found the boys, who told me that if peeing in public was good enough for that semi-conscious woman over there it was good enough for me. I was seconds away from disaster so I tore off down a residential side street and ducked into the first dark driveway I found. There were people coming along the street but I was beyond caring. I squatted down and did a wee of bovine proportions, watching as a small river of urine snaked down the driveway towards the closed garage door.

Suddenly the strip between the garage door and the driveway lit up: someone was in there – as, by now, was a growing puddle of hot piss. Even when the garage door started opening I couldn't do anything to stop peeing, but when a burly bloke emerged, effing and blinding, I grabbed the crotch of my jeans – still peeing – and lolloped, Quasimodo-style, down the street as I struggled to pull them up.

One of my newfound friends was so charmed by this performance that he ended up asking me out. We now have two young minds of our own to corrupt.

I grabbed the crotch of my jeans – still peeing – and lolloped, Quasimodo-style, down the street as I struggled to pull them up.

French farce

CAITLIN B.

When I was sixteen I signed up for a Summer Abroad scheme in France, along with a bunch of other American teens who had rarely or never left the States. While most of them opted to spend a month in glitzy Paris or the sunny Côte d'Azur, I with my romantic notions of Europe told the scheme's organizers that I wanted to go 'to the countryside'. And so it was that I was packed off to a farm in the middle of Christ-knows-where to stay with a family in which nobody spoke English.

The family consisted of two parents and five sons aged between sixteen and what seemed pretty ancient at the time but was probably about twenty-nine. The eldest two sons were the ones who'd signed up for the exchange programme at the French end – and coincidentally or otherwise the two who seemed happiest about adopting a naïve sixteen-year-old American girl for the summer – so I spent most of my time with them, miming my pleasure or displeasure at whatever they mime-suggested we do. Our communication woes were so dire that we spent most of our days cycling around the nearby fields and hills so as not to have to speak.

One day the eldest son, Luc, suggested a bike ride and I happily agreed, grateful for an excuse to burn off some of the cheese and unidentified meat products I had been force-fed since my arrival. It had got to the stage where I would have killed for a tomato or even just a couple of grapes. I threw on my school gym shorts and a T-shirt and off we went.

We hadn't got very far before the exercise began to have the previously desired food-burning effect – so much so that I was doubled over my handlebars with stomach cramps on the flat stretches and actively clenching to avoid shitting myself on the hills. At one point I had to get off my bike just to focus on keeping everything in. Luc looked concerned and asked if I was alright – I assume that's what he was saying – and I mimed 'Feeling a little rough – will battle bravely on,' before jumping back in the saddle and pedalling off with a fixed grimace.

By the time we got back to the farm I knew I was beyond
saving: something entirely awful was about to happen.
I leapt off my bike before it had even come to a standstill
and was about to run inside when Luc raced up and asked
what was wrong. I was fine, I assured him, although by now
I was twisting and tightening the ends of my little shorts so
that they'd contain the shit that my bowels no longer could.
He kept asking what was up and I just couldn't get away.
Suddenly my face, and perhaps the terrible smell, must
have explained everything. It was happening.

I ran away as fast as I could with my hands trapped by my
thighs, only letting go when I reached the stairs up to my
little granny flat. Warm shit streamed down my legs and over
my shoes as I waddled up to the bathroom. I was in there for
an hour or more and nobody came to check on me – they all
knew I was otherwise occupied.

Many hours later, when the mother knocked tentatively
at my door to ask if I'd like any dinner, I mimed 'Never
eating again.'

'Probably for the best,' she mimed back, and disappeared.

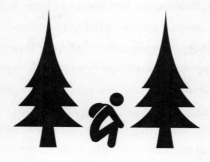

If you go down to the woods today . . .

ANDREW W.

One summer, when I was six or seven and visiting family in the middle of nowhere in Canada, my cousin and I went on an excursion in the woods. We climbed trees, played Cowboys and Indians and pretty much ran around screaming for a couple of hours.

At one point in the afternoon, both of us realized quite suddenly that we needed to poo. This is never an issue in the woods as there is rarely anyone about and Mother Nature provides an abundance of suitable material for the after-event clean-up. One does need to be careful not to select the wrong plant, however, as there are a few large-leaf varieties that cause a burning sensation followed by extreme itchiness. We went our separate ways on either side of the woodland trail and our respective number twos passed, so to speak, without much drama.

We were within hollering distance of each other and just as I had finished and was wandering back to our trail I heard loud exclamations of unsavoury vocabulary coming from the bushes my cousin had chosen. Assuming he must have picked the wrong kind of leaves I ran and grabbed the right kind and rushed through the undergrowth to save him.

I found him standing behind a bush with his shorts pulled up and a great quantity of shit on his feet and legs. It turned out he had crouched, pooped and wiped without issue, but then pulled up his shorts to discover he'd crapped directly into them.

Wetsuit

VICKY A.

Last summer, my boyfriend and I went on holiday to
Australia with a couple of other friends. We'd taken the
opportunity to go on a scuba diving trip with a number
of other holidaymakers.

Given that I was fifteen metres below sea level and in a
wetsuit, I figured that letting out a surreptitious fart would
easily be concealed by the bubbles from my breathing
apparatus. And yet, something felt decidedly dodgy about
my stomach that day. It was only as we got back onto our
boat that I grew concerned over that unmistakable smell.

As I unpeeled my wetsuit in full sight of the rest of the
group, my fears were realized when it was confirmed that
I had, in fact, shat myself. It was all down the inside of
the wetsuit, and now on my hands. My boyfriend and
friends will never let me live this story down – made more
excruciating by my own disbelief as I offered a shit-covered
hand to the horrified stranger beside me on the boat and
said, 'Look what I've done.'

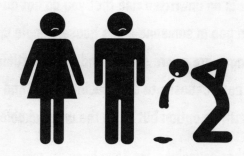

PART TWO:
UNWELCOME GUESTS

It is an unwritten rule that you do not do a poo in someone else's house. People of all ages are aware of this, and yet sometimes your body chooses to defy social mores, and leaves you with no option but to do the unspeakable.

On other occasions, we have been warmly welcomed into someone's home and shown wonderful hospitality and kindness. And then the booze takes hold and we forget where we are, making us reverse all good will with one sticky hand print on the wallpaper . . .

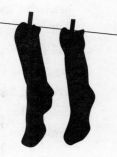

Sock story #2

ADAM G.

A bunch of us went to stay at a friend's parents' place
in the country for a birthday weekend last summer.

When we arrived, I was shown up to my bedroom by
our friend's dad, who was the house-proud type: pictures,
rugs and god-knows-what-else were all pointed out to
me on my way to the room.

The boozing started straight away, and by the end of the
night I was several dozen sheets to the wind. I passed out
in my room in the early hours.

In the middle of the night, I woke up with a crashing headache, and an unwaivable urge to go for a shit. I was still completely pissed, and the room was pitch black, so I stumbled around for a while trying to find any sort of exit. It was a total failure. I couldn't see a thing, couldn't find a fucking door, and I started to freak out. In my drunken desperation, I hit upon what seemed to me a rather genius idea.

I picked up my used sock from the floor, held it open and shat into it. I then flung the very offensive item out of the window.

When I woke up the next morning, drunk and confused, I could immediately smell that something had gone horribly wrong. Imagine my complete and utter horror as I gradually became aware that the walls and ceiling were spattered in shit. I then saw a brown smear down the window – and the soiled sock in a heap on the carpet below.

Not only had I failed to open the window before trying to throw the sock away, but I had evidently also held the wrong end of it as I flung it across the room.

Something like Cinderella

<u>SAM C.</u>

During the Easter holidays of my first year at university, a friend invited a whole bunch of us to his parents' house out in the suburbs for one of those debauched weekends that always ends in tears and vomit. I didn't disappoint on the vomit front; my friend's mother provided the tears.

It was the last night of our stay – the parents were due back in the morning – and we had given the house a thorough clean before getting pissed and negating all our good work. I have no idea how the party ended but the next thing I knew I was lying in my sleeping bag on the living room floor and I had an overwhelming urge to puke.

The lights were off and the house was silent, so I crawled out of the sleeping bag as quickly and quietly as possible, ran down the corridor and vomited in the toilet. I cleaned myself up pretty well, stumbled back down the corridor, and went back to sleep.

I woke up with the worst headache of my life, knackered, confused – and covered in puke. The living room stank. I had no idea what time it was or where my friends were. Just then the door nudged open and the family's small dog wandered in. It took one horrified sniff of the room before retching into a nearby shoe (mine).

I had to get out of there before I added to the already considerable puddles of vomit, so I staggered out into the hallway and navigated my way to the bathroom by the pukey handprints that lined both walls. I got in there to find my friend's mum frantically scrubbing the carpet. Sensing that this was no time to engage her in a debate about the wisdom of laying carpet in a bathroom, I mumbled an apology, grabbed my things and walked four miles to the train station. In one shoe.

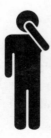

I have no idea how the party ended but the next thing I knew I was lying in my sleeping bag on the living room floor and I had an overwhelming urge to puke.

Meeting the parents

ADAM G.

I went to my girlfriend's parents' place a couple of years
ago for Sunday lunch. It was the first time I was meeting
everyone, so I was pretty nervous. Her dad spent the first
hours grilling me about my life plans and ambitions, but her
mum was kind, her grandmother was polite, and I had met
her two sisters before. All in all, it was going pretty well.

We sat down for lunch in their conservatory, and after
the starter I used the pause in the meal to go to the loo.
My girlfriend gave me a quick smile as I left the room, to
indicate it was all going well, and her mum pointed me
towards the bathroom upstairs. Once I was there, I realized

I needed a crap, and thought I could get away with making it a quick one before heading back downstairs.

Without going into too much detail, this one was a corker. I was already taking a bit longer than I'd wanted, so rushed to finish up and head back down. I was about to leave the bathroom when I saw that the fucking thing hadn't flushed properly, so I waited for the cistern to refill and gave it another go: this shit was not budging.

I could hear my girlfriend's mother plating up the main course downstairs, and I began to become agitated. What was worse: leaving a massive shit in their loo when the next person to use it would know it was me, or missing lunch because I was too busy trying to flush the toilet? I was panicking, and knew I had to act quickly.

In a split-moment decision, I wrapped my hand in toilet paper, grabbed the solid turd from the bowl and made a shit parcel. Still a little unsure of what to do next, I heard someone downstairs say, 'Oh, well let's just start without him,' as they tucked into the main course. I had to act now!

Without thinking, I opened the bathroom window and threw the turd out, hoping it would land in some bushes by the house and go unnoticed. I flushed the loo once more for effect, and nonchalantly stepped downstairs and into the conservatory.

The room was silent, and everyone was looking busily down at their plates. My girlfriend's face was blushing and her sister had a smirk she was trying to disguise. They must have been wondering what on earth I was doing in the bathroom for ten minutes. Then my girlfriend darted a look at me, and then up at the ceiling.

I looked up, and sat in the middle of the conservatory roof – directly over the dining table – was my solid shit covered in strips of wet toilet paper, which must have landed with a splattering thump just as they started eating.

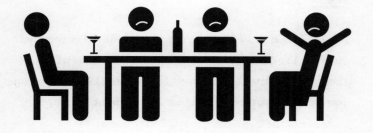

Darling, can I come in?

ROB

My girlfriend and I took the plunge and moved in together last year. We'd reached that stage in a relationship where there are very few mysteries left about one another, and you want to share everything. Or so I thought.

One evening, I came home from work and had – quite frankly – needed a crap since I left the office. As I entered the house, I could hear from the splashing of water that she was having a bath in our one and only bathroom, and so I shouted hello through the door and thought I would wait it out. But no matter how much I busied myself about the house, the urge to go to the loo would not abate. There was no avoiding the fact that this was going to happen in the next minute, whether I liked it or not. And so with the hugest apologies, I opened the bathroom door and headed straight for the toilet, repeating, 'Sorry, sorry, sorry!'

It was only as I sat down and emitted a torrent of shit that I noticed the scented candles, the glass of red wine on the side, and the low relaxing music that was blighted only by the sound of my arse. The look of disbelief on my girlfriend's horrified face told me I had well and truly trampled her vibe. Through the ensuing yelling, I gleaned that she had been having a terrible week at work, and was not best pleased with her one hour of down time being interrupted by the sound, and smell, of my shit.

I had learnt my lesson; the forty-eight hours of frosty reception saw to that. And yet, about a month later, I found myself in exactly the same position as I entered our flat: desperate for a crap, but with my girlfriend clearly in wind-down mode in the bathroom. Fuck. There was no way I could make the same mistake twice.

After pacing the flat, changing out of my suit, trying to sit down, stand up, pacing again – anything – I still was absolutely in dire straits. A number of options presented themselves, each more ridiculous than the last, and sadly none of them involving a toilet. I cannot stress enough how imminent the need to crap was.

I grabbed a plastic carrier bag from the kitchen and went out into our patio. Could I actually shit in my own garden? I had to stay close to the wall of our house so that the neighbours couldn't see me from their first-floor windows, and lowered my trousers around my ankles, squatting indecently over the bag.

The lasting memory of the incident is of our pet dog sitting in the kitchen, staring out at me through the patio door with a perplexed look on his face. He tilted his head, appalled by my behaviour, before he turned and walked away.

Welcome home, darling

KATH W.

It was the summer holiday between my first and second years at university and I was back at my parents' house in the suburbs, being sullen and lazy and an all-round drain on resources. My older sister was there too and we spent our first night home knocking back bottle after bottle of prosecco and setting the world to rights while our parents went to bed.

It must have been about 2.30 a.m. by the time we staggered upstairs, but I was awake again at 6. I had this overwhelming feeling that I needed fresh air. I got up and went to my window but it was locked – my dad had evidently shut and sealed my room when I'd gone off to university. I stumbled into my parents' room and flung open their window, then leaned out of it gasping loudly. Unsurprisingly, they woke up.

'What the hell are you doing? [etc., etc.]'

'Blrrgh,' I told them, and then made a dash for their en suite bathroom. I suddenly knew that I had to get some nebulous evilness out of my system.

I was sitting on their toilet, both parents cautiously tapping on the door and asking if I was quite alright, when I felt a strange cold tingling at the top of my head. Slowly the feeling began moving down my scalp, past my eyes – which blacked out – and then my ears – I went deaf – and I only just managed to fumble blindly out into my parents' bedroom before I fainted. And then I shat myself and vomited on their carpet.

The postman never rings twice

JOE G.

After a swanky black-tie work party, one of my colleagues
decided it would be a brilliant idea to continue the festivities
back at his. It was already about 1 a.m. on a Wednesday
morning but we were beyond caring about having to go
to the office in a matter of hours.

I can't remember much of what happened in his flat – pizza,
music, whatever alcohol we could get our hands on – but
by around 4 a.m. everyone else had left and my host was
passing out on the sofa. I felt it was time to be sensible and
go home. I let myself out of his flat into the corridor that led
to the main entrance of the building. His front door had just
slammed shut behind me when I remembered there was a
special key for opening the main door, and I obviously didn't
have it. Inevitably, I suddenly needed to pee.

I went back down the corridor and knocked on my
colleague's door. No response. I banged harder – nothing.
I called his name and thumped with both fists, but he was
clearly in an alcoholic coma on the sofa. I went back to the

main door and peered through the letterbox, hoping some passing gang of youths might be willing to kick the door in for me, but the street was silent.

I spent the next two hours sitting at my colleague's door, periodically banging my head against it and cursing his name as the horrors of my hangover washed over me. The birds were singing outside by the time my need to pee got the better of me. I knew there was no hope of rousing the sleeping bastard and that I had lost my last shred of dignity by finding myself drunk in a dinner jacket three hours before work, so I wandered back down the corridor and, praying that the postman wasn't coming up the garden path at that moment, peed out through the letterbox.

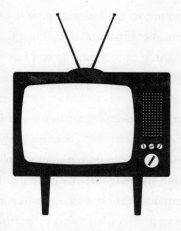

Top of the poops

CLAIRE S.

When I was fifteen I used to hang around with this girl called Michelle, not so much because we had lots in common and enjoyed each other's company but rather because I fancied the pants off her brother Ben. He barely knew I existed but that didn't stop me from going round to her house at every opportunity to watch TV while pouting seductively, or do my homework while flicking my hair about.

One evening I'd gone over to watch *Top of the Pops* and Ben was in charge – the parents were out – so naturally

I was making quite an exhibition of myself. During a Boy George number I had a sudden terror that my mauve eyeshadow might need touching up so I sultrily slunk off to the bathroom.

I have no idea what possessed me to make myself quite so at home while I was in there, because obviously it's against every social rule to poo in someone else's house, and especially within smelling distance of someone you fancy, but the fact remains that I did a huge turd and couldn't make the bloody thing flush. I tried twice, three times – and then realized there are only so many times you can pump the flush without raising suspicion. If I didn't get back out there before the top-ten countdown they'd know something

I tried twice, three times – and then realized there are only so many times you can pump the flush without raising suspicion.

was up. Obviously there was no question of just leaving
the turd there: if Ben saw it he'd never marry me.

There was a pack of toilet rolls in the corner so I stacked
the contents in a neat pyramid and fished the turd out using
the plastic bag. Now what?

I stuffed the soggy package in an inside pocket of my
handbag and, obviously not before the all-important
announcement of that week's number one, took my
number two home on the bus with me.

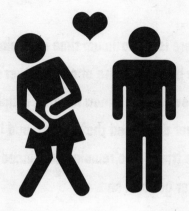

PART THREE:
DATES
FROM HELL

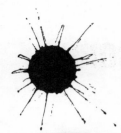

There is no optimum time in a relationship to become aware of one another's bowel movements. I know married couples who have never discussed the subject, and I have one male friend who remains convinced that girls never go for a shit.

And yet sometimes it is unavoidable. There is something thoroughly excruciating about the dating scenario, in which we try our hardest to display our very best qualities and yet accidentally end up displaying our very worst attributes. All over the bed, in some cases.

Do you want to come in for a coffee?

SARAH

A couple of years ago, I went on a first date with a guy I met online. We went out for dinner and were having a really lovely time together.

Halfway through the meal, just as I was beginning to think this could really go somewhere, I started to feel a bit unwell. I styled it out for a while, and was able to carry on with the dinner for as long as I could. But before the desserts arrived, my stomach was already making weird noises and I couldn't hide it anymore.

I didn't want him to think I was doing a runner, but I absolutely had to get out of there at once. He could see that I was genuinely feeling under the weather, and like a gentleman he offered to walk me home. But it was on the way home that things took a turn for the worse. I started to feel really dodgy.

I picked up the pace a bit, and I know I was talking at double speed just to distract myself. We finally got to my front door, where our first kiss was a panicked peck as I scrabbled around in my bag for my door key.

It was dark and I was frantic, and I just couldn't find my keys anywhere. I could sense that something truly hideous was about to happen ...

I rang the bell for my flatmate to let me inside, all the while trying as best I could to maintain my share of the polite end-of-date chitchat. What happened next was reported back to me after the event.

My flatmate came to the door and said an awkward hello to my date. At which point, I took one step into the flat, vomited onto the carpet, and fainted on the floor into my own sick. I then promptly shat myself at their feet.

Perhaps alarmingly, I am now married to this man.

Wind beneath her wings

DAVID G.

I was woken up suddenly in the middle of the night by an
excruciating thirst. I opened my eyes and could not for the
life of me remember whose house I was in. I recalled being
in a bar with friends, doing shots of tequila and chatting
to any girl that would listen. And now here I was, in a dark
bedroom I didn't recognize, and absolutely parched. One
certainty was that I was still completely pissed.

I glanced over to the other side of the bed, and in the
darkness I could make out a female body. Result! She stirred,
and could see my eyes were open.

'Come here,' her voice croaked.

I still couldn't remember who the fuck she was, but I wasn't
about to pass up an opportunity like this, so kindly obliged
her advances before we both passed out.

'Mummy!'

This was the shout that woke me up again in daylight. What the fuck? I scrabbled for the duvet to cover myself just as a lively child ran into the room, said something unintelligible about cereals and ran out again. I looked over the bed again – this time in excruciating daylight.

She was the size of a house, evidently the mother of several children, and with a habit of bringing random men back to the family home. She turned her head to look at me. Oh god. Her face was puffy and glistened with grease. Seeing her with last night's make-up smeared and her damp hair stuck to her face, I suddenly felt yesterday's tequila rising up again. I ran to the bathroom and was sick in the toilet.

When I emerged, I could hear she had gone to get the kids their breakfast. I had to get out of there. I threw on my clothes that had been strewn across the floor, picked up my bag, and cautiously tiptoed down the stairs and towards the front door. I couldn't bear the idea of bidding farewell, so scrabbled at the various locks of the door to get out.

'Leaving so soon?'

She had found me. She planted a wet kiss on my lips, leaving the taste of cigarettes and coffee to mix with the taste of vomit I already had. She unbolted the door for me, and I walked shakily down the front path into the bright daylight.

I closed the gate behind me and turned to wave goodbye. She stood in the doorway in her dressing gown and with a fag hanging out of her mouth. With a wry smile, she lifted the front of her nighty to show me the treasures I had delighted in only hours before.

That was it. The sight of her growler was more than I could handle: I steadied myself on the gate, vomited immediately on her garden path, wiped my mouth clean and left without a word.

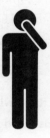

With a wry smile, she lifted the front of her nighty to show me the treasures I had delighted in only hours before.

Going down

TOM P.

A few years ago, I started dating a girl. We'd been out a few times, and the moment finally came for us to spend the night together for the first time.

We were having good fun back at my place, and at one stage I started to go down on her. All was going smoothly, and we both seemed to be enjoying ourselves, when she suddenly let out a small fart. Not wanting to make her feel awkward, I just laughed it off – and she started to giggle with embarrassment.

I continued to do what I was doing down there, when suddenly her giggles made her lose all control and she quite simply crapped in my bed and on my chin.

We both froze in complete disbelief and excruciating embarrassment for a moment, before she made a very swift exit via the shower amid hurried and mumbled apologies.

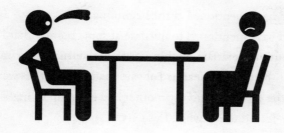

Lovely to meat you

LIAM J.

After I left uni and moved to London, a friend of mine
set me up on a blind date with his girlfriend's cousin. He'd
been banging on about her for ages and I'd seen a couple of
really pretty photos so I was quite nervous. We arranged to
meet for dinner and I let her choose the restaurant on the
pretence of being gentlemanly – in fact I didn't have a clue
where cool young Londoners hung out. When I arrived at
the designated spot it turned out to be a Korean restaurant,
which as you can imagine were few and far between in
my hometown of Carlisle in the 1980s, but my date was
stunning and I was up for a culinary adventure. I gamely
ordered a No.23 with a side order of No.56, choosing them

solely because the only word I could understand in the descriptions was 'vegetable'.

I should have mentioned at the beginning of this story – as I should have mentioned to my date at some point – that I'm vehemently vegetarian. Nothing to do with ethics, I'm afraid; just that the taste of meat had always made me barf (as we said in the eighties), and my mother had given up trying to force-feed it to me when I was six.

As you'll have guessed by now, my meal, when it arrived, was basically a plate of unidentified flesh swimming in a vegetable mulch. I literally have no idea what it was. It smelled, to me at least, like Gandhi's flip-flop, and looked like something that had been regurgitated.

'Mmmm!' said my date, looking over at my food.

'Yummy,' I replied unconvincingly, backing up my appraisal by swiftly sticking a forkful of the gristly matter into my mouth.

I knew immediately that I'd made a terrible mistake. My guts contracted once, then twice, and I felt whatever was in my stomach beginning to well up like lava. I still had the meat in my mouth and I emitted a sort of squeak that alerted my date to my distress. She looked at me in terror.

'Oh my God, are you choking?'

Before I could respond she'd called over three waiters who arrived just in time to watch the mouthful of meat fly across the table at her, followed by a stream of semi-digested lunch, which, I had time to note, rather resembled the stewed vegetables on my plate.

Credit where it's due, at least my date didn't run out of the restaurant screaming. It was more of a sobbing shuffle, while wiping her dress with napkins.

Wet dream

BELINDA D.

Back at uni, my long-term boyfriend and I had been out
drinking at a boozy student party. I hasten to emphasize that
we were both considerably shitfaced. After the party, we went
back to my room for the night and promptly both passed out.

I had one of those awful dreams where you are going to
the toilet, and it became quickly apparent that I was indeed
pissing the bed in real life. I woke up first, but my movements
made my boyfriend stir as well. Completely mortified,
and horrified at what he would make of this, I woke him
with a jolt and shouted, 'Oh my God! Darren – what have
you done?'

To this day, he still believes it was he who wet the bed
that night.

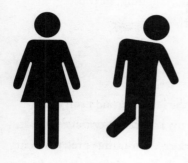

Have a nice life, yeah?

JAKE F.

My new girlfriend and I had been dating for a month and everything was going great. We spent every spare moment together and were very much in that 'blinded by love' phase where you're convinced the other can do no wrong – and where you want them to think you can do no wrong, so you're both on best behaviour.

One sunny Saturday we went up to Hampstead Heath with a picnic and wine. It was such a lovely afternoon, marred only by our first instance of 'bad' behaviour when I accidentally burped during lunch.

'Oh my God,' my girlfriend said, laughing, 'next thing we know we'll be farting in bed.'

If only.

We were on our way home in the late afternoon sun when I felt an unpleasant stirring in my bowels. Fortunately her flat was only about ten minutes away and I was pretty sure I could hold it in – but the knowledge that there wasn't far to go actually seemed to make it all worse. I really needed to poo. It got so bad that I even had to utter those three little words for the first time in our relationship: 'I'm gonna shit.'

My girlfriend laughed nervously, thinking I was exaggerating, but I knew something terrible was about to happen. I started desperately looking for a pub or cafe or someone's front garden I could go and squat in, but it was no use. I was going to have to make it back to her place

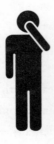 **'Put loud music on!' I yelped as I shuffled towards the toilet, trying unsuccessfully to contain the mess in my jeans.**

somehow. By now I was walking like John Wayne and clutching my stomach, sweating as I tried to concentrate on my girlfriend's attempts to take my mind off things, and when we eventually reached the front door I seriously considered just letting it all out and then dealing with our inevitable break-up.

I gave up all pretence of decorum as I half-waddled, half-crawled up to her bathroom, undoing my jeans as I went – and I nearly made it to the loo! No sooner had I flung the bathroom door closed behind me than I lost all control of my bowels and, frankly, shat everywhere.

'Put loud music on!' I yelped as I shuffled towards the toilet, trying unsuccessfully to contain the mess in my jeans.

I was in there for the next half an hour, scrubbing, showering, lighting scented candles, wondering how and where to incinerate my clothes, and mentally composing my online dating profile.

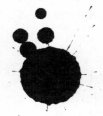

I love you, too

PHIL S.

I had been dating a guy for a few months, and we had gone on a boozy date one weekend. Drinks, followed by dinner, followed by drinks, followed by cocktails, followed by a nightcap back at mine. Needless to say, we were pretty hammered and having a great time. Feeling the full force of the booze, I don't think we even finished the two glasses of whiskey I didn't even know we had in the house, and we went to bed.

We embarked on an approximation of sex, and I remember thinking that he was unusually quiet. I translated this as the manifestation of some deep emotion – that our sex had moved from pure lust to something more sensual. I looked at him with all the soulfulness I could muster and said in a soft tone, 'I think I'm falling in love with you.' He looked me in the eyes with a gaze that said he really understood me.

Or that's what I thought it was.

We were still, er, very much in the middle of things and the motion must have stirred up those last few drinks, because he clumsily lurched to his side and was promptly sick over the edge of the bed and onto the carpet.

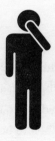

We embarked on an approximation of sex, and I remember thinking that he was unusually quiet.

First impressions

ROBERT G.

Last year, I had met a new man at a friend's birthday party and we quickly hit it off. Within a week we had been on a couple of dates, and the following week he invited me to the house party of a friend of his. It seemed a little soon to be meeting all of his friends, but we had been having a great time together and I was keen to make a good impression. Needless to remark, I was not successful.

As we approached the house door, I let my date go ahead and climb the three steps up to the doorbell. I stayed back, suddenly identifying this as one of my last opportunities of the evening to let out a small fart. But something awful happened: at the very moment that the door opened and we were greeted with a smile and cheer, I shat myself.

Oh fuck.

Not a full-on pant-fill, but enough to make it the most uncomfortable social occasion of my life. With what must have been a strained grimace on my face, I limped into the house. Within one minute I was greeted by twenty different people, all of whom I was trying to ensure liked me, while at the same time waddling around nervously like a weirdo and terrified that I stank of shit.

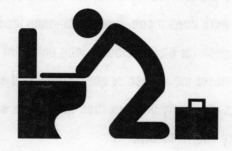

PART FOUR:
WORKPLACE
DISASTERS

It is a universally accepted fact that no one at work does a poo. Even if someone leaves their desk for a suspiciously long period of time, it is never mentioned or questioned, and everyone looks nervously down at their keyboards when the guilty culprit returns.

So in this setting, what happens when you are inadvertently caught short? To avoid admitting that you are doing the unspeakable, it becomes necessary to hide all tracks — sometimes literally — of your actions. And all of this while wearing a power suit and trying to maintain an air of professional capability.

Hovering hell

NATALIE H.

I had just started at my current job, so this is a couple of years ago. During the day, I went into the bathroom near our desks, and did what any proper lady does and hovered over the seat as I went about my business.

When I'd finished, I immediately realized that somehow, while in the hovering position, I had actually shat into my own knickers and onto the inside of my skirt.

I froze. I could feel the heat from my own face as I wondered what the fuck I was going to do next.

The knickers went straight into the sanitary towel bin. I made vain efforts to scrape what I could off the inside of my skirt with some toilet paper. When I was sure the bathroom was silent, I darted out to the sink to moisten some paper, and scurried back to the cubicle to scrub my skirt again, but it just seemed to exacerbate the problem.

By this point, I was a wet mess. The only item in my bag that could begin to help was a tube of roll-on deodorant, which I promptly applied all over myself and the skirt. I waddled nonchalantly back to my desk, worried that they were about to send out a search party for me.

I could do nothing but sit down sheepishly at my desk, with a drenched skirt, no underwear, and stinking of shit.

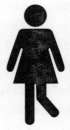

I waddled nonchalantly back to my desk, worried that they were about to send out a search party for me.

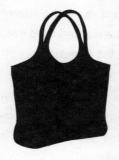

Handbags at dusk

ANNABEL G.

I was out with colleagues one Thursday after work. As happens on such occasions, 'one drink' at the end of the day had turned into quite a session. I had an important client to meet on the Friday morning, but had nonetheless been very easy to convince into staying on 'til the bitter end.

So much so that I had no hope of catching the last train home, and accepted the offer to stay at a colleague's flat – after one last drink, of course. By the time her and I were finally ready to leave the bar, I was feeling beyond pissed.

Once seated in the back of a taxi to her place, the spinning interior made me decidedly nauseous. As the car traversed London at speed, every turn seemed to hasten the inevitable. I was too embarrassed to ask the driver to stop in the presence of my colleague, and tried to concentrate on getting to the end of the journey.

I was not successful. The sick rose instantly and there was no time to do anything rational – I opened my handbag and noisily puked over all its contents: my purse, keys, phone, scarf and make-up.

Knowing I'd have to wear all the same clothes the next day, my pissed mind had the foresight to wash the scarf in the sink when we got to her flat, and I wore it for my meeting the following morning.

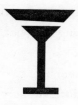

One reason I hate jazz

ANDREA

One of my colleagues was celebrating her thirtieth birthday and had hired a table at a cool jazz club in London's Soho on a Saturday night. I didn't know her that well but she'd invited everyone from the office and was really excited, so I decided to go along. Inevitably, I was the only person from work who showed up, an awkward situation I attempted to alleviate by drinking myself into a stupor.

With a few unidentified cocktails inside me, I was starting to feel at one with the music – never a good sign – but at the same time the saxophonist had apparently turned into three people, all of whom were swaying across the stage. It wasn't long before the room started spinning backwards.

I intuited that this augured ill. I tried to focus and get back into conversation with the strangers at the table; in between hiccups I bellowed something no doubt intelligent-sounding at the girl across from me.

'Um, sorry,' she interrupted after a short while, 'but you've got a leaf or something on your face?'

It took me a while to find the mystery object, and then to focus my eyes on it, but it looked suspiciously like a morsel of chewed-up spinach, last seen going into my digestive system at lunchtime that day.

With a sense of hideous foreboding I looked down. Oh, fuck. The scooped neck of my little black dress was full of vomit, now swilling around as I tried to stand up.

'I think I just puked,' I wisely declared, before stumbling down to the toilets and passing out until well after closing time. I never thought I'd be so pleased to be poured into a taxi by a couple of cleaners rather than by the people I'd spent the evening with.

Shopping shocker

KATY M.

I was on my way into work one morning with a stinking hangover, and nipped into a shop to buy a birthday card for a colleague. I'd had a restorative cigarette on the way, which in hindsight may not have been the most prudent idea.

The bright lights and patterned carpet of the shop were doing nothing for my mood, and as I neared the counter, I began to feel decidedly nauseous. Steadying myself on the till, I asked as politely as I was able whether I could possibly use the staff toilets very briefly.

'Oh, no – I couldn't possibly let you in there,' came the clipped response.

Before I could register this, I had taken a step back, and promptly vomited everywhere. And I mean everywhere: on the side of the counter, across the nearby merchandise, and in a huge splat on the floor. There was a moment when the two of us just stood there – she with a look of frozen horror on her face, and me hunched over with vomit dripping from my mouth.

Having lost all sense of what was going on, I reached to the counter to grab a large paper gift bag – with no absorbent quality whatsoever – and vaguely wiped my face. I mumbled an apology and said something about cleaning it up. To my disbelief, the shop assistant agreed entirely, and noisily went to get me the cleaning equipment.

So I found myself on all fours, wearing rubber gloves, and scrubbing at the carpet in the doorway of a card shop on the way to work, thinking my life had hit its lowest possible point. And then:

'Katy? Is that you?'

I turned to see two old school friends standing in the doorway of the shop with pitying and puzzled looks on their faces. All I could do was hopelessly point at the wet soapy puddle and say, 'I just did that.'

And they left me to it.

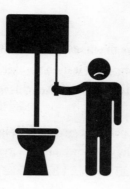

Lights, Camera...
Oh, no...

HANNAH M.

When I was starting out in television production, I spent a couple of months temping on a TV drama. We were filming in a large suburban house just outside of London, and being the young newbie, I had to be on set watch while the rest of the crew took their lunch break. Fairly quickly, I'd finished my own packed lunch, had flicked through the dog-eared newspapers, and still had twenty minutes before everyone else was due back on set.

I rolled up one of the newspapers under my arm and took myself up to the first-floor bathroom to make the best use of my time. It was only after I'd done my business that I realized

I'd made a very grave mistake. I pulled on the chain hanging down from the cistern, and it didn't budge. I took a closer look at the toilet. My heart sank. Yes this was a prop toilet.

Two things were apparent: first, my colleagues were all coming back from lunch in fifteen minutes to film a scene in this bathroom; and second, I had a fake toilet full of shit.

The silver lining around this very dark cloud was that it was at least fairly neat. This meant I could use half of the newspaper to scoop the offending turd from the bowl, and then wrapped it all up in the remainder of the paper. I tiptoed down the stairs holding the grim parcel, praying that no one had come back from lunch early.

I couldn't bear the thought of the owner returning to her house after we'd all packed up to find an awful stench coming from her bin, so the only way to dispose of the package with a clear conscience was to throw it in the open bin bag we had next to the crew's tea urn and hope for the best.

I spent the rest of the afternoon as we filmed upstairs in a complete panic that someone would mention the smell of shit coming from the bin, or the fact that the toilet looked like it might have been used . . .

All rise

STEPHEN L.

I'm a barrister, so most mornings I find myself on a train
leaving London for a courtroom somewhere in the south
of England. It's a very traditional profession, and a smart
appearance is everything. You don't want a bewigged judge
to glare at you from the bench for having an unstarched wing
collar or for wearing the incorrect day-of-the-week socks.

On one morning journey, I paid my regular visit to the train
loo, and sat down with my daily newspaper. Hearing the
noise of some people outside waiting to use the cubicle,
I was conscious of not stinking up the whole carriage when
I was done – so I decided on a mid-loo flush to help clear
the scene. If you ever find yourself in a similar situation,
I recommend that you do not remain seated when activating
the flush.

The force of the vacuum flush sent a sploosh of brown water
up the front of my pristine white shirt, down onto the inside
of my suit trousers, and – well – all over my balls.

'Fuck.'

I did what I could with disintegrating toilet paper to soak up the water from my suit and shirt (and undigniﬁedly from between my legs), but it had left clear brown marks on anything it touched – most visibly on my shirt. I was getting hot and agitated wondering what on earth I could do. Squirting soap from the dispenser onto some toilet paper, I proceeded to work a brown lather into my shirt, only making the situation more horrendous by the second. It took me the remainder of the train journey to get anywhere near sorted, and I darted out of the cubicle and waddled onto the platform in my wet trousers as soon as we reached the stop.

I walked into court and had to immediately give off a professional air. I approached the man whom I was responsible for keeping out of prison today, petrified that at any point he would realize that I was in fact covered in my own shit.

Tubular smells

LISA

I'd been out for a colleague's leaving drinks on a Thursday night, and it had turned into a horribly late one. The following morning, I found myself staggering down to the London Underground and making my way to work with a colossal hangover. In fact, with my hair in a state, my bloodshot eyes barely open, and my shirt unironed, I'm not entirely sure that I wasn't still pissed.

I stood on the crowded platform and already felt stifled by the musty warm air of the tube. As a train approached, the draft made me sway slightly, and I seriously wondered whether I should crawl home and call in sick. The throng of people pressed towards the opening train doors, and we crowded in.

I was squashed against the side of the carriage, surrounded by warm bodies, men's armpits and that musty smell. The train rocked from side to side, and the taste of last night's Sambuca was swimming in my warm mouth. I had a brief horror that I was going to be sick right then, and realized I had to get off at the next stop no matter where it was – but by the time we reached it, I managed to contain myself somewhat and thought I would brave it all the way to work.

Oh God, if only.

The train set off again, and the musty Sambuca warmth returned. The bright fluorescent lights combined with the constant prod from the moist belly of the man behind me and I was overwhelmed – I suddenly realized I wasn't going to be able to keep it in this time. An involuntary belch made everyone's heads dart my way. I was going to be sick. Now.

I held my hand over my mouth in a naïve attempt to hold anything back, but I could feel it coming up. In a split second I had a choice: to projectile vomit all over a crowd of already displeased commuters, or somehow to contain the imminent disaster. In an instant, I turned right round to my left to try to throw up in the corner of the train, and instead was noisily sick into the coat hood of the man standing with his back towards me.

'Oh fuck – I am so sorry.'

The next three minutes were a slow-motion blur of insufficient apologizing, horrified faces, and one very confused man. We stood on the platform of the next station briefly with him shaking out my vomit from his hood, and me vaguely saying something about dry cleaning. He held his coat with disgust, but seemed to genuinely understand how mortified I was. As the doors beeped to signal the train was on the move again, he jumped back on and was gone.

I stood on the platform, hunched over, wondering how the fuck I was going to get back home.

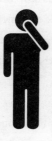

The next three minutes were a slow-motion blur of insufficient apologizing, horrified faces, and one very confused man.

Blame game

<u>HARRIET</u>

I was working in an office where at least fifty women had to share two toilet cubicles – the thin-walled sort where the partition doesn't reach to the floor or ceiling and you are always very aware of sitting next to your boss with your pants round your ankles. You could practically admire each other's shoes while peeing.

Anyway, I'd gone in one day for a simple pee and found the bathroom empty. I was about to lock myself into one of the cubicles when I noticed the most enormous shit in the toilet bowl. Now, we've all heard the phrase 'enormous shit' before, but, seriously, it is impossible to overstate the size of the fucking thing. The notion that it had ever emerged from a dainty lady is, to say the least, eye-watering. I wisely dashed into the other cubicle.

It was only while washing my hands that a terrible thought struck me: if anybody comes in right now, or sees me leaving and then comes in, *they might think it was me* ... It was too terrible to contemplate so I resolved to finish what the rogue pooer had started. But just as I leaned into the cubicle and put my hand on the flush, the bathroom door started opening behind me. In panic I locked myself in with the enormous shit. Someone else's enormous shit.

I could tell from the overwhelming perfume and the jangling bling that the new arrival was our MD. I had to get out of there ASAP. I pressed the flush a couple of times in the hope that the cistern would appreciate the magnitude of the challenge ahead. Nothing happened. I mean, water sloshed about a bit but the poo remained wedged.

Now I was in a bit of a pickle. The MD was centimetres away from me, pants round ankles, and I was locked in a cubicle with an unidentified shit that wouldn't budge. If I left right now there was every chance I'd be back to square one re copping the blame. Worse, in fact, since anyone coming in would have to take my cubicle. I started sweating. There was only one thing for it: I was going to have to wait this fucker out.

The MD left eventually, no doubt wondering why someone who'd flushed the loo was still just standing there in silent contemplation, and I flushed with all my might: nothing. Again: nothing. People came and went. I flushed: nothing. Nothing! Not a fucking quiver. It was like trying to flush a Subway sandwich.

At this point I began to seriously consider climbing out of

the tiny window and taking my chances on the six-floor drop. I had been in there at least fifteen minutes. I started panicking about which client I could possibly charge this to on my timesheet.

Finally, in weary resignation, I knew it was time for the endgame. It was me or the poo, brain vs brawn. I took a deep breath and grabbed the toilet brush. This was not going to be my finest hour but at least I had a weapon. Then, in a frenzied scene that'll be filmed in extreme slow motion in the movie of my life, I smashed that fucker up. It was like something out of *A Clockwork Orange*.

It still took two flushes to get the damn thing down but my nemesis was finally vanquished. Sweating and dishevelled, I emerged wild-eyed from the women's loos and spend the afternoon sizing up my colleagues for likely culprits.

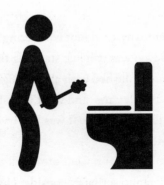

A splash in the pan

LAUREN H.

It was 10 p.m. and I was at work, pissed. As a single twenty-something with a very junior job in the media, you can imagine the enthusiasm with which I threw myself into the spontaneous drinking sessions that cropped up on the most spurious of pretexts. I have no idea what we were celebrating on this particular occasion but the drinks trolley had been finished off and security were telling us to get the hell out before they locked up for the night.

My friend Pete and I said we'd walk to the tube together and both went off for a final wee in the reception toilets. I suddenly realized I was absolutely bursting. I found the women's toilets in complete darkness and couldn't find the light switch anywhere – there were no windows either – but as I'd used this bathroom every day for the past couple of years I reckoned I could manage it in the dark. I felt my way to the cubicle, closed the door and then shuffled backwards towards the toilet. Aha – there it was! I pulled down my jeans and went in for a ladylike 'hover'.

I was about five seconds into what promised to be a record-breakingly long wee when I noticed I was getting a surprising amount of splashback from the bowl. I must not be in quite the right position, I thought, shifting around a bit. It didn't help; in fact things seemed to be getting worse. About eight seconds in it suddenly dawned on me: the toilet lid was down. There was no chance of stopping mid-wee so I quickly reached round and lifted it up.

Ptsssssssch! A torrent of piss cascaded round my ankles, all over my flip-flops – incidentally, I was wearing flip-flops – and started working its way up my jeans. The whole cubicle was swimming in about a centimetre of urine. I stared helplessly into the darkness.

When I'd finally finished weeing I could turn my attention to panicking. What the hell was I going to do? For all I knew it was seeping under the door. I unravelled the whole roll of toilet paper and threw it about me, sloshing around in the flood as I tried to get into every corner. I gathered up the soggy bundles and flushed what I could but I had no way of surveying the remaining damage. I had to escape.

I squelched out to the sinks, my flip-flops suctioning to the floor as I went, and washed my hands. A lot. Then I casually wandered out of the building to where Pete was waiting. Fortunately it was dark enough and he was drunk enough not to notice that I looked as if I'd been wading.

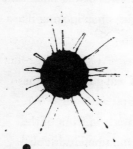

Fashion faux pas

PAULA M.

During my gap year I went to work in one of London's swankiest department stores. I had zero customer-service skills and the money was terrible, but it kept me out of trouble. More or less.

In the run-up to Christmas the management announced that there was no budget for a proper staff party. Instead we would have a fashion show and treasure hunt in the store, with lashings of booze and an inadequate number of canapés. All the young people were rounded up in advance and informed that they – this included me – would be the fashion-show models. We were given priceless but fusty old-lady clothes to wear and spent an hour each in the make-up department having our faces put on. There were so many of us taking part that my make-up session was before lunchtime and I had to go out to the local sandwich shop looking like a geisha in a business suit.

But I digress. Once the last customers had gone, the wine came out, and my friends and I went at it with gusto. We were really nervous about having to parade in front of the senior managers in expensive clothes and uncomfortable shoes, and by the time the music started we were all trashed. I have snippets of memory from my tour of the 'catwalk' – snaking in and out of the pillars and chairs in what I no doubt assumed was a seductive fashion – but the next thing I knew I was in the pub.

You could still smoke in pubs in those days and my boss was puffing away rather glamorously. Clearly, I thought, this was my moment to develop a new grown-up addiction, so I grabbed the fag out of her hand. I'd only inhaled a couple of times before I realized how incredibly drunk I was; light-headed from the smoke I got up and staggered to the tube.

Somehow I made it to the London terminal from which my train to the suburbs left. I had to wait for the platform to be announced and I recall slumping against a wall with my skirt round my thighs and my face a mess of purple eye shadow and smeared lipstick. I knew by the time I got on the train that I was going to be sick – a prediction that unhappily came to pass just moments after the doors closed when I vomited on the seat beside me.

I called my dad to come and pick me up from the station and finally got home to find a scene of domestic normality – parents chatting over wine, siblings watching *Friends* – into which I crashed, stumbling and incoherent, and looking as if I'd been out paintballing. It was the first time my mother had seen me drunk so she was, to say the least, a little alarmed when I tripped my way up the stairs and shut myself in the bathroom.

The glorious final scene of this mortifying drama had me sitting on the loo and suddenly needing to vomit. I turned around without pulling my pants up, crouched over the loo and was sick once again – just as my parents and wide-eyed little siblings threw open the door to make sure I was OK.

The only good thing that came out of all this is that, fifteen years later, I still can't even hold someone's cigarette for them without feeling nauseous.

Fingerlickin' bad

RACHEL T.

I was at a work picnic one sunny day a few years ago. We'd
been reluctantly herded out of the office to the nearest park
and were sitting by a big lake with little boats and geese and
the like, and people were playing rounders and Frisbee and
generally having a surprisingly fun time.

Everyone had brought a dish or two, so the buffet area
was pretty impressive. I loaded my plate up with various
unknown bready things and dips and went to sit down
with my colleagues. A few minutes later I was holding court
in an animated fashion about the previous night's reality
TV when I saw I had a blob of olive tapenade on my finger.
I licked it off. I am told my face suddenly resembled that
of 'a dog licking piss off a nettle'. It was not olive tapenade.
It was goose shit.

People always interject at this point in the story and ask,
'How did you know it was poo?' – to which the answer is
that I just did. You would too. There must be some innate
knowledge in the human palate of what poo might taste
like. I'll save you some effort right now by saying: not great.

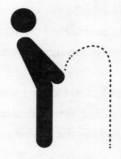

Alight for Waterloo

ANDREW D.

I'd escaped my work Christmas drinks as soon as was decent and dashed to the nearest station. But in my haste I'd failed to go for a safety wee at the pub, and as a result I was now facing the very real prospect of pissing myself on the tube.

I sized up my fellow travellers. It was still only 8 p.m. – dark outside but very bright in the carriage – and most them were just sober commuters on their way home to a lovely evening. Unlike your average 11 p.m. crowd, they'd probably notice if I had a quick slash in the standing area. Bollocks.

There were still six stops to go until mine, and at each one I desperately tried to remember if there was a nearby pub at ground level, but whenever the doors opened I just couldn't trust myself to move without letting it all out. By the time the train approached my station it felt as if I was on the verge of rupturing a number of vital organs.

As we pulled in I knew I was done for. The doors opened and I hobbled out – followed by a few dozen commuters – whipped out the old lad and pissed against the side of a passenger bench on the platform, muttering over and over: 'I'm sorry. I'm sorry. Oh, God, I'm so sorry . . .'

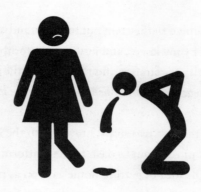

Pulling a sickie

GARY M.

I work in media, and in the summer we take any opportunity to pop to one of the pubs near our office for a delicious lunchtime pint in the sun. On one such occasion, I had remained relatively well behaved and only had one pint before returning to the office to get on with some work. I picked up a sandwich on the way and ate at my desk.

Within half an hour of returning, I started to feel decidedly dodgy. I knew I couldn't be pissed, and wondered if there had been something odd with the sandwich. Suddenly thinking about it made my stomach twist. I made my way to the bathroom and sat in a cubicle groaning slightly for about twenty minutes before resolving to make my way home.

I slouched down in the train out to the suburbs, holding my head down by my knees, and just waiting for the journey to be over. I felt very strange and the speed of the passing city made my head spin. *I must not vomit, I must not vomit.*

At each of the first two stops, I toyed with the idea of leaping out of the train to dash to the platform toilets to be sick – but the idea of getting home as soon as possible was all I could focus on, so I remained there cradling my head in my hands. We then reached Clapham Junction, and the carriage filled with people, even though it was a Thursday afternoon. I suddenly felt trapped, and hot, neither of which sensations was helping with my churning stomach.

This is it. I'm going to be sick.

I could feel the warm saliva filling my mouth. I was at the point of no return, and needed to make a dash for the train doors before they shut again. I called for all the busy commuters standing around the door to get out of the way – or at least that's what I wanted to do. Instead, I didn't want to risk opening my mouth too much and made a muddled grunt as I signalled with my hands for them to move. 'Myurgh.'

I took two steps from where I was towards the door, and immediately lurched forwards and was sick. On the floor, on a man's suit trousers, and on the feet and high heels of one horrified woman. On her fucking feet. For a moment I stood hunched over, while trying to utter the words, 'I'm so sorry.'

The mumbling of my speech as my stomach still convulsed and the evident aroma of beer from my vomit made them all assume I was just pissed in the middle of the afternoon – so just as the doors beeped to signal their closing, I was unceremoniously shoved out of the train with a boot and a venomous 'Fuck off!'

I slumped down on to the platform, with vomit down my chin and sobbing lightly, wondering how the hell I was going to get home.

Merde

<u>BETH P.</u>

As part of my degree course in French I was packed off
to a small town in southern France for a year to earn my
keep as a highly inexperienced and wholly unenthusiastic
English teacher. My charges were eight years old and I was
completely useless at controlling them, never mind imparting
my supposed wisdom on the subject of grammar.

One rainy Monday morning I was in a particularly foul
temper and the prospect of asking thirty-three little bastards
to regale me with tedious tales of *le week-end, en anglais s'il te
plaît*, was entirely awful. We'd only got through three of them
when my classroom nemesis, Jean-Luc, put his hand up and
asked if he could go to the loo. Perhaps because of my mood,
or just because he needed to learn, as I had fifteen years
earlier, that asking to be excused brings out the worst in any
teacher ('Can I go to the toilet?' 'I don't know . . . Can you?'),
I wheeled out that other timeless teacher classic: 'You should
have gone when you had the chance.'

He whinged for a while until I yelled '*Non!*' – which
strangely actually shut him up. He seemed awed by my
uncharacteristic adherence to common classroom rules.

I forged on with my weekend round-ups but Jean-Luc was forever in the corner of my eye, unnervingly quiet and increasingly pale. Just as we got to his turn the boys on either side of him leapt up dramatically and announced over the top of each other that Jean-Luc had let one rip. The whole class burst into screeching hysterics and all the kids within ten metres of him shuffled their chairs away, claiming they were trapped in a cloud of fart.

We were within three minutes of the end of the lesson so I said everyone could stay where they were as long as they shut up and listened to Jean-Luc's story. And so it was that all eyes turned to him, sitting alone in the middle of the room, just in time for the unmistakable sight of the poor boy shitting himself. He went bright red, emitted a sort of strangulated bleating and burst into tears. I pretty much did likewise, minus the poo.

The other kids were looking at me in a sort of panic, waiting for me to do something suitably grown-up. I'm mortified to say that the first person to break the silence was Jean-Luc, who said, through his sobs, and in perfect English, '*May* I go to the toilet?'

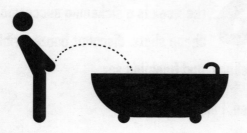

PART FIVE:
STUDENT
CATASTROPHES

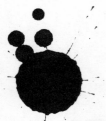

Students are disgusting. Every night of the week is a sickening succession of cheap shots, discount booze, dribbling kebabs, and fumbling sex.

God, I miss university.

It is the first time in our lives that we are treated like adults, and the last time in our lives that we can behave like children — a wonderful mixture of no responsibility and the ability to drink. It is this heady cocktail that leads to some of our most reckless behaviour and most revolting memories, hazy though they are.

Fight Club

JAMES P.

A few of us were having a boozy session in a busy pub back at uni. Our mate Steve had a bit of a reputation for being the first to suffer from overindulgence, and he soon began to look unsteady on his feet. His face turned pallid and he started to sweat, so he quickly took himself off to the pub toilet as we got another round in.

About a minute later, he came running out of the toilets like a man possessed. He looked me straight in the eye and said, 'We have got to leave now!' and pushed his way outside at speed. Seeing that something really serious had just happened, we left our pints and chased after him into the crowded street.

Through his panic he told us how he had rushed to the toilet to go and be sick. He had taken the scenic route to the gents, zigzagging and stopping to hold on to things, and by the time he got there his face was green and he was on the verge of vomiting into his own hands.

Knocking past the guys at the urinals, he bashed through a cubicle door, lunged forward and was sick – right into the lap of a massive bloke who was having a shit. The bloke roared and recoiled as best he could (Steve had landed with one hand on the cistern and the other on the man's bare thigh) and they paused there motionless for what felt like minutes, each more incredulous than the other at this horrific scene.

Steve staggered to his feet, wiping his hands on the walls and trying to focus his eyes. He made the split-second analysis that he was about to get punched – and so he swung forwards and pre-emptively smacked the poor guy right in the face.

He then turned and ran away.

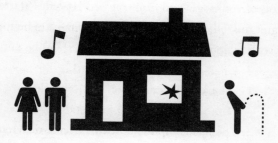

Pink Kangaroo

LEWIS P.

When I was at uni, I fancied myself as a bit of a DJ and would offer my services to any friends having a party – with the understanding that I would then not need to bring any of my own drinks for the night. At one particular party, I'd been on the decks for most of the night, and took a break to let someone else have a go.

Being a true host, my friend could see that I had some catching up to do with the booze, and so made me what he called a Pink Kangaroo. He was as hammered as everyone else, and I wanted to join in. He half-filled a pint glass with cider, and followed that with a slug of blackcurrant cordial.

He grabbed the nearest bottles from the table and poured in shots of vodka, gin and rum – at which point I started to regret the folly of agreeing to this tipple – and he topped it off with lemonade.

'Why is it called a Pink Kangaroo?' I naively asked.

This is when he picked up the bottle of Crème de Menthe, and dropped a shot of it into the pint. It promptly curdled as it passed through the cordial, and created what could be described as an upside-down pink kangaroo floating in the cider (if you were pissed enough and squinted your eyes).

Even as a student, I could see that downing this in one go was not going to end well, so I instead spent an agonising fifteen minutes nursing the hideous mix – each layer more undrinkable than the last. Soon enough, the desired effect had taken hold and I was an unstoppable force at the party.

Toward the end of the night, and innumerable drinks later, I wasn't doing so splendidly. I had somehow managed through my increased confidence to hold the attention of a girl for quite some time, and even though I must not have been able to string a sentence together, she seemed to be returning my flirtation. At some point, I lurched in for a snog, and we stood in a clumsy embrace for a moment.

As I shut my eyes, the room started to spin. The taste of cider on her breath was all too familiar, and the memory of chewing through the curdled Crème de Menthe was making an ugly return. I could feel the Pink Kangaroo wanting to make an unexpected reappearance.

Mid-snog, I gave the poor girl a forceful shove away from me, and simultaneously hunched over and vomited on her legs.

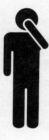

He grabbed the nearest bottles from the table and poured in shots of vodka, gin and rum – at which point I started to regret the folly of agreeing to this tipple.

Hide the poo

OWEN D.

In my second year at uni, I moved into a student home with three other male friends. I feel that I should preface this tale with an explanation that we were revolting young men. Our level of banter had reached absurd heights during our first year of juvenile freedom, and culminated in one of the most horrendous displays of indecency, which I am secretly quite proud to have been involved in.

I forget whose idea it was, but during our inaugural drinking session in our new home, one of us introduced the game of 'Hide the Poo'. The rules probably don't require much explanation, but we were all tasked with concealing a turd somewhere in the apartment, with the winner being the owner of the last one to be discovered. Over the course of the next few hours of drinking, each of us slunk off to the bathroom to do our thing, while the others continued boozing on my bedroom floor. By about 2 a.m., one of the most hideous games of hide-and-seek ever had begun.

The first two were quickly found on that same night: a suspicious plastic bag behind the sofa, and my rather meagre clingfilm parcel in the bathroom cupboard. The third turd took until the next evening to reveal itself, but only because the sandwich box containing it had been concealed at the back of one of our cupboards behind a little-used vacuum cleaner. This left the final offering somewhere in the house, and our new cohabiter Nick keeping completely tightlipped regarding its whereabouts, only convulsing in fits of hysterics whenever we pressed him.

Life moved on and we deemed the game to be over. Nick was crowned the winner a couple of days later, and we forgot all about it. It wasn't until a week after we moved in that the hideous hiding place was made apparent.

While getting ready the following Monday morning, our housemate Jarrod went to the kitchen to make a quick tea and toast before heading out to his lectures. He boiled the kettle and buttered his toast. And as his knife scooped through the butter, a layer of brown was revealed. Nick had actually removed the soft butter from its plastic container, and placed his turd underneath before concealing it again with the butter – and it had then been sitting in our fucking fridge for a week before Jarrod spread it on his toast. Nick's title as winner of the game was very well earned.

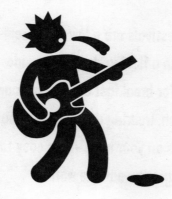

PART SIX:
FESTIVAL FUN

Festivals are a law unto themselves. Lost in a field in the countryside, drinking beer for breakfast and eating magic mushrooms for lunch, wearing day-glow face paints and teeny boppers on your head — it's easy to see how you can forget the outside world.

No one around you has had a shower in days, and the toilets are a fucking disgrace. But in your pissed haze, lying in the sun and surrounded by like-minded lunatics, nothing could be more perfect. Until you lose control of your bodily functions.

Fun guy

BETH

I was at a huge music festival a couple of summers ago
with a big group of friends. One of the guys in our extended
group had been talking the whole weekend about getting his
hands on some magic mushrooms, which he eventually did.
Fairly soon after munching a handful of them, he started to
act quite spectacularly strangely, but we were all enjoying the
music and left him to his own wonderment as he wandered
through the crowd.

Several hours later, we saw him again in the distance, holding
his hands out at people with a beaming smile on his face.
I could see one group of people he'd found himself with
looking horrified at him, with one of the blokes telling

him quite distinctly to fuck off. So we sent two of our male friends over just to check he was ok.

It turns out he had been sick into his own hands, but was hallucinating so madly that he thought he had vomited pound coins instead of sick. He had his coat pockets full of the stuff and was generously handing it out to the crowd in glee.

When our two friends finally caught up with him, he was at the bar, incredulously arguing with the barmaid about why she had a legal requirement to accept his tender.

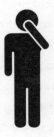

He had his coat pockets full of the stuff and was generously handing it out to the crowd in glee.

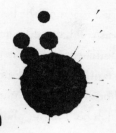

Shock horror

AMY

Last summer I went to Glastonbury, and after several years of slumming it in the mud, a friend and I resolved to spend the extra cash and hire one of their on-site caravans for the weekend. This gave us unprecedented luxuries like electricity, our own toilet cubicle and even a shower, not to mention a guaranteed dry bed.

What it did not do, however, was help in any way with the horrendous hangover of each day. On one particular morning, I opened my eyes to gauge my whereabouts: I was in our caravan in the blistering heat of the late morning sun. I sat up blearily and looked around to see my friend lying in an awkward position across the other half of the bed. I let out a small belch. Sambuca.

Oh God. My stomach started to convulse.

I tried to get off the bed to dash to the toilet cubicle, but I was still half asleep and my legs were tangled in the sheets. I launched my body over my friend's sleeping lump, and was instantly sick off the side of the bed – and immediately saw I'd been sick on the multi-plug socket in the wall from which both of our phones were charging.

In my hungover brain, I managed to compute that electricity and vomit was probably not a good combination. So without blinking I grabbed the plug to get it away from the wall, and immediately was jolted up by an electric bang followed by that familiar smell of burning hair. My friend sat upright in an instant and shrieked, 'What the fuck happened?!'

'I electrocuted myself with my vomit.'

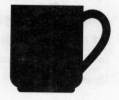

I wouldn't drink that

PENNY D.

A few summers ago, a group of us returned to Glastonbury, and I brought my boyfriend along for his first festival adventure. Having sold it to him as a wonderful summer experience that would change his life, I'm glad I was right on at least one count. The rain did not stop pouring all week, and had turned the whole area into a wet and muddy hell, and the event became a survival situation even for those of us who were festival veterans.

During the day, we would stomp about in our wellies and rainproof ponchos, but would fairly quickly be wet through to the bone in our cold, wet jeans. At night, we would return to the tents as late as possible to peel off our clammy clothes and huddle together in our sleeping bags.

One night, I lay in the sleeping bag hearing the rain drizzle down, and could only think about how much I needed to pee. I turned from side to side hoping I could sleep, but the need just got worse. There was absolutely no way I could get my damp clothes back on to march through darkness to the toilet area, and yet something had to be done fairly immediately.

I quietly wriggled out of my sleeping bag in the pitch black, desperate not to wake my boyfriend, and very, very slowly unzipped the inner door to the tent. I was paranoid that each frantic jerk of the zip would wake him. I got myself into the small porch area, squatting over his tin camping mug and pressed against the wet outer layer of the tent.

As I sat there piddling into his cup, I was sure he was lying awake in disgusted silence, and all I could think was, 'Well, this certainly is a new low.'

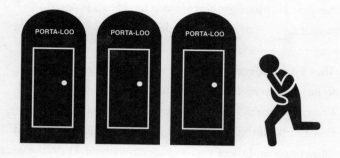

Festival toilets

MATT

Festival toilets are notorious for their grimness. When you're at a music festival for a few days, though, there is simply no way of avoiding them. I was with a few friends at Bestival on the Isle of Wight, UK a few summers ago, and we'd spent the whole day wandering from one bar to another, drinking beer in the sun. We went back to our tents in the late afternoon, already considerably hammered, so we could stock up on our own drinks for the evening.

I took this juncture in the day to stagger off to the nearest bank of toilet cubicles for the inevitable daily session. The queue was consistently about thirty people long, no matter what time of day you went, and so I stood at the back swaying ever so slightly from side to side and waited my turn.

The closer I edged towards the cubicles, the closer I was to needing to relieve myself. Finally it was my turn, and I ran to the cubicle, sat down and went. It was only then that I noticed the empty toilet roll holder. I looked around desperately and there was no paper anywhere. With the next shower a few days away, this was a hideous situation to be in.

Even though it was certain there would be paper in one of the other toilets, there was no way I could waddle out in front of the waiting crowd and start knocking on the other doors for some help. This was awful! I looked around the small plastic cubicle for some inspiration – any inspiration – but found none.

Realizing I was in a terrible predicament with very few options, I started to unlace one of my trainers. Still completely pissed, I proceeded to unsatisfactorily wipe my arse with a shoelace, which was very quickly rendered useless. With a sigh, I leant forwards and undid the second shoelace and achieved what I could.

I plodded back towards our tents with my loosened shoes and an ashen face, prompting immediate concern from my friends. When I told them what had just happened, one friend bent double with laughter and asked, 'What's that?' as he pointed at my shorts.

Sticking out of my back pocket was half a roll of toilet paper that I had taken with me to the loos.

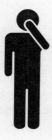 **Still completely pissed, I proceeded to unsatisfactorily wipe my arse with a shoelace, which was very quickly rendered useless.**

PART SEVEN:
BOOZY
EMBARRASSMENT

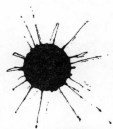

Booze has a lot to answer for. It is the reason why we're all slightly fatter than we want to be, why we look four years older than we think we ought, and why you have that child you weren't expecting. Oops.

The great thing about booze, however, is that any regrettable behaviour or ghastly situation can be explained away the following day with an apologetic, 'Sorry, I was really pissed.' It provides the perfect excuse for behaving with a complete disregard for social norms and allows us to tell people exactly what we think, even if we've already said it five times that evening.

And wearing traffic cones on our heads will always be funny.

Kebab house horror

JEREMY P.

Only a few weeks ago, I spent a boozy day in the pub with
friends. We'd gone for a quick pint in the early afternoon,
and it ended up being an unexpected all-day affair. After
we'd finally been booted out of the pub at closing, we went
our separate ways home.

Having eaten nothing other than nuts and crisps all day,
I stopped off at the kebab house round the corner from my
flat. The last beer was catching up on me, and I quite urgently
needed a piss, but ordering a portion of chips and cheese was
more important to me at that moment. As they cooked my
order, I started to jiggle from one leg to the other to help
prevent myself from pissing all over the kebab shop floor.
I thought I was being surreptitious about it, but I must just
have looked like a shitfaced guy who needed a piss.

Suddenly I could take no more, and asked if I could use
their staff bathroom. I think I blurted out the question really
abruptly, and one of them showed me downstairs into their
one basement cubicle. The release of being able to piss was
a huge relief, but that emotion was to be brief.

I let out a small fart, and immediately froze: I had in fact just shat myself. It was only a small amount, but enough to be of quite some concern. Because this was their staff toilet, and they were probably already waiting upstairs with my order, I didn't feel that I could embark on a clean-up operation right there – so instead just zipped up and waddled awkwardly back up the stairs.

The two-minute walk back to my flat from the kebab house was amongst the least glamorous moments of my life: hungrily shovelling cheesy chips into my mouth, while shuffling along the street with pants full of shit, and hoping desperately I didn't accidently crap myself again before I reached my front door.

Beer belly

TOM G.

Two friends and I had got tickets for an international beer festival in London. It was a Tuesday night so we'd vowed not to sample too many of the thousands of delicious foreign ales available but, well, there were thousands of delicious foreign ales available. Not one of us can remember leaving.

The next day at work we were all feeling rather sorry for ourselves and comparing notes via email. It turned out that, while we had no recollection of stumbling out of the exhibition centre, we had all had regrettably memorable nights. One of my friends had woken up covered in vomit, the other had woken up to discover he had somehow broken his ankle and needed to be taken to hospital, and as for me . . . Oh dear.

I'd taken the tube home and was crashing down my road, banging into cars and walls on either side, when the gallons of beer inside me began to take their inevitable laxative effect. But I was so close – just another five minutes and I'd be home – so I clenched and played 'I Spy' with myself to take my mind off things . . . Car, cat, recycling box, massive heap of dogshit – lucky dog . . .

It felt like ages but then, like a mirage, it hove into view: my house! I made it! I'm home and dry!

Oh.

My elation, and indeed my bowels, suddenly got the better of me. I just shat myself. I was so stunned that I actually just stopped and stood there outside my house, warm shit running down my legs and into my shoes, unable to compute what the hell I was supposed to do now. I could see my girlfriend in the front room, watching TV. Awkward.

Eventually, I took one shuffling step forward, then another, each movement encouraging more solid matter to slide southwards into my socks. I let myself in and called out that I was just nipping to the loo, with you in a sec, and then raced upstairs to the bathroom. I was in there for half an hour. My jeans, pants, socks and shoes were write-offs; I bundled them all into a plastic bag, showered, and found some clean clothes in the airing cupboard.

I emerged, dry and warm, still pissed, and pretty impressed with myself, all things considered, clutching a bag of shitty clothes, to find my girlfriend furiously scrubbing brown stains out of the carpet. She's a keeper.

The only way is Essex

KELLY P.

Many years ago, a group of us girls all went out for a night on the tiles in Basildon. We were just out of school, and would spend most of our Saturday nights together in one girl's house, applying fake tan, getting the eye lashes mounted onto our clown-like faces, and backcombing our hair with half a can of hair spray each. Our sense of fashion wasn't much better: each in the highest stilettos that prevented us from actually walking more than five metres in one session, and a variety of brightly coloured and revealing dresses.

We all thought we looked stunning, but looking back at the photos now is excruciating. We were only about eighteen years old, but looked like thirty-five-year-old drag queens doing fancy dress. On this particular night, I was wearing a tight-fitting white mini dress and heels that made me walk like Bambi.

We'd had a fair amount to drink at home, tanking up beforehand so that we wouldn't have to spend too much money in the club. Inevitably, we then also spent loads of money in the club on drinks – with luminous alcopops following electric blue shots following Sambuca. At some

point late on in the night, I tottered uneasily towards
the ladies toilet, holding onto the wall to steady myself
on the stilettos and booze.

Once in the safety of the toilet cubicle, I held onto the sides
and lowered myself into the 'lady hover' with my mini dress
hoiked up around my waist. Without going into too much
detail (too late), I went for a poo. I grabbed some toilet paper
to wipe my arse, but as I did so and let go of the wall, one
stiletto wobbled to the side, and I slipped down onto the seat.

Brown shit stain all up the back of my white dress.

There was absolutely nothing I could do – any attempt to
rinse it off would have made my tiny dress not only more
brown, but entirely see-through. Despite what you might
think, this is not the sort of thing that is acceptable in Essex,
so I rushed out into the reassuring darkness of the club and
demanded that all the girls hide me as I made a hurried –
and teary – exit.

Gin and gin

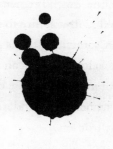

GREG R.

The first time I discovered gin was at a house party when I was at school – I must have been about sixteen years old, and had no concept of my limits. I hated the taste of alcohol back then and, after a few courage-building drinks, I realized that doing large shots of the stuff tasted just as horrible as sipping it slowly and yet was over in a fraction of the time. So that's what I did. I have recollections that still make me shudder today of my friend Sam creating a new cocktail for me.

'It's called a Gin and Gin,' he slurred, as he thrust a tumbler into my hand and half-filled it with gin.

After a pause, he considered the glass and said, 'Right – you're gonna want to have some gin with that,' and filled the second half up from the same bottle, gin sploshing onto my hand. 'Now, see it away.'

The consequences of that cocktail were inevitable, so I'm not sure how much I remember, or how much I remember being told ... But suffice to say that I needed considerable attention, something that a gaggle of useless teenage boys was unable to provide in an adequate fashion, and it wasn't long until my parents were called. They found me lying in the garden next to a puddle of vomit, and pukey mud stains all up my trousers.

My parents took me home, placed me slouched on the stairs, and embarked on the sticky task of undressing me in the hallway. I can clearly recall advising them that I'd quite like to go to the bathroom – but in hindsight, this must have emerged from my catatonic face in a series of mumbled grunts. The next thing I hear is my mother's voice.

'He's shat himself.'

They dragged my limp body to the bathroom for an industrial hose-down, and called an emergency doctor. His diagnosis was that I was, indeed, pissed. I spent the night on a makeshift bed in my parents' bedroom being monitored for signs of life, and woke up feeling very sheepish the next morning.

Whenever I went out for the next year-and-a-half, my mother would say to me, 'Enjoy yourself – but not too much,' before giving me a wink. Fifteen years later, I still cannot touch gin.

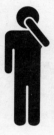

They dragged my limp body to the bathroom for an industrial hose-down, and called an emergency doctor.

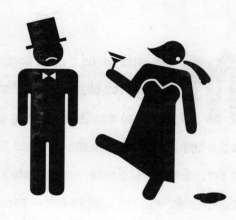

PART EIGHT:
NICE DAY
FOR A WET
WEDDING

Many girls spend a good portion of their young lives planning The Perfect Day. From the wonderful flowing dress, to the beautiful venue, to the canapés that will be served, the first dance, the speeches, the bridesmaids, and the honeymoon — everything is regimentally choreographed to a strict image.

And this is all before they even have a boyfriend.

Sadly, things don't always go the way they are planned, and very occasionally the most anticipated — and most photographed — day of your life becomes a miserable nightmare.

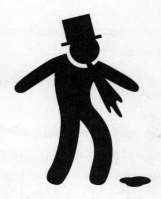

Worst man

PETE M.

Last summer, my longest standing friend Mark got married. We have been friends since school, and so it was the clear choice that I would be his best man. His fiancée's family is religious, and so they held the ceremony in a gorgeous country church near her family home.

Despite the event certainly not being all about me, I nonetheless felt progressively more nervous when the big day arrived. We had done a rehearsal of the ceremony the evening before, and all went well – but for some inexplicable cause, the day itself made me very nervous. I think it was seeing all the friends, families, grandmothers and whoever else from both sides all coming together for one big day of

events, and knowing that I was partially responsible
for making sure nothing fucked up.

I was unsuccessful.

We'd spent the morning getting ready with Mark and the
rest of the ushers, and now stood at the front of the church
as it filled with the congregation. I had huge sweat patches
under my arms that I could hide beneath my suit jacket, but
my clammy palms and nervous flush were less easy
to conceal.

When his fiancée began her agonizingly slow walk down the
aisle, it was as though I grew more nauseous with each step
she took. I steadied myself on the groom while pretending to
give him a supportive pat on the back. I had a mental word
with myself to pull myself together and get through it, even
if I was sure I could feel those few glasses of champagne
from earlier bubbling in my stomach.

The priest's sermon droned on interminably. His words
made both my eyes and my stomach swim. I remember one
of the ushers looking over at me and mouthing, 'Are you
ok?' I had to get some fresh air. If I could just breathe cold,
fresh air, I would be able to dash back in time for the actual
marriage bit.

Without a word, I discreetly scurried down the side of the church and out of the main door. I saw a couple of concerned looks from the congregation in my peripheral vision, but kept my eyes down as I trotted out. The air hit me, and within one step of exiting the church, I hunched over and vomited clear champagne into a bush on the side.

I stood there, stooped over the bush and thinking how I would shortly rejoin the ceremony as if nothing had happened. Simultaneously, I'm told the priest had had to stop his sermon mid-sentence as the sound of retching echoed around the building, punctuated only by a reverberating 'Oh, fucking hell'.

Lady in yellow

PAULA D.

I got married six years ago in the spring. I wasn't a complete
bridezilla, but I had spent about fourteen months from the
point we got engaged planning the big day. From the cake,
to the venue, to the dress, the dinner menu and the music
– I had a very clear idea how I wanted the day to go.

Sadly, things don't always go to plan. The dress I had chosen
from the scores I tried on was a gorgeous fitted number
with satin ribbon up the back and it kicked out at the base.
It was – like many things – slightly over the original budget,
but I easily convinced myself it was worth it.

On the day, I'd spent the morning getting ready with my
girlfriends. I didn't want to peak too soon, so paced myself
with just one glass of champagne and plenty of water as I
had my hair and make-up done, and then got into the dress
while the bridesmaids readied themselves. The car arrived
and we all gathered by the door ready to go, when I suddenly
thought I should go to the loo before I leave – who knows
when the next opportunity will be?

I was suddenly aware of all the water I had been drinking

over the past couple of hours. The car was ready, we were all about to leave – and I now desperately needed a piss. I asked one of the girls to help me, but everything seemed to take twice as long in a wedding dress: placing the bouquet carefully down somewhere, shuffling past all the bridesmaids in the hallway, walking sideways up the stairs one step at a time. By this point it was becoming an emergency. I think I was screaming.

I flung off my heels and hurried down the corridor to the bathroom, dutiful maid of honour in tow. I could barely walk in the figure-hugging dress, let alone run. Inside the bathroom, the panic went up several notches: 'How the fuck do I get out of this dress?' My voice was shrill.

I was grappling with the base of the dress, my maid of honour was trying to carefully undo the satin ribbon down the back, and I was becoming sweaty and agitated, jumping from side to side. And then it happened. I actually pissed myself in the most expensive thing I've ever bought. It was only a partial piss, but enough to precipitate more screaming and involuntary tears, as I was eventually able to break free and land with a piddling thump on the toilet seat.

I was never able to explain to my now-husband and to all of our family and friends why I turned up to our wedding quite so late, but spent the rest of the day convinced that everyone I spoke to thought I stank of piss.

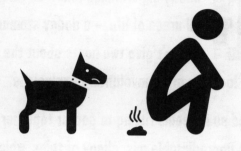

PART NINE:
ODDS
AND ENDS

Ghastly experiences follow us through all areas of life — a dodgy stomach doesn't give two hoots about the time or location of its involuntary explosions.

And so it seems fitting to gather together here an unpredictable miscellany of tales, which otherwise defy categorization.

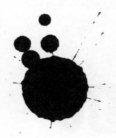

Let's farty!

GRAHAM P.

One of the major perks of having a teenage sister is that they regularly bring attractive young girls to the family home. When my little sister was about nineteen – I was ten years older than her – she and a friend tried their hand at fashion design, as part of which they put on a pretty professional catwalk show followed by a boozy celebration for all the scantily clad models back at our house. Clearly my brothers and I and everyone we knew offered to be on hand to maintain order.

The music was blaring, the alcohol was flowing and it was all going swimmingly when, out of sheer giddiness, I went to fart on my friend Dave – quietly and imperceptibly, you see, so that only he would notice. Instead, I full-on shat myself. I'm talking the entire contents of my bowels all over my legs and even down onto my feet. Of course I was in the very middle of the room full of girls.

The only thing I could do was waddle as unnoticeably as possible – which, as discussed, was not at all unnoticeably – to the bathroom, where I threw my trousers and underwear out of the window and took a shower before re-emerging in non-shit-stained clothing to continue my flirting campaign.

I slept alone that night.

Midnight confession

HARRY G.

After a few months of travelling in South East Asia
I had taken a circuitous but relatively cheap series of
interconnecting flights home to Canada. It had seemed
a good idea at the time, but it ended up taking about
thirty-six hours and I was completely shattered and pretty
disorientated by the time I finally pulled into my darkened
driveway. It was after midnight when I got in so I resolved
just to go to bed – but, oh, look, a few cans of Guinness in
the otherwise empty fridge. It would have been rude not
to toast my safe return, so I drank a couple of cans and
then went upstairs.

I had just got under the sheets and was easing myself into
sleep mode with a few Guinness-inspired farts when I did
one that was rather explosive and wet. I zombie-shuffled
to the bathroom to clean myself up, but there was no toilet
paper. I went to get in the shower, but the water was still
shut off from before I went away.

So down to the basement I went with a torch and a shitty
arse to find the water valve. I was pretty sure I knew where it
was: under the basement stairs at the very back of a narrow,

pipe-filled cubby hole barely big enough for a cat to get into, let alone a fat bastard like me. In I went, flashlight in mouth, shit rapidly drying at the other orifice, in search of the elusive valve. I couldn't find it. I checked every corner of the cupboard and it simply wasn't there. I was basically out of options: no toilet paper, disconnected telephone, no shops open and no fucking water. I decided to just sleep on my stomach and deal with it in the morning.

The next morning I walked to the nearest payphone – which of course was in a mall – with an asscrack full of dried shit, to phone my brother and ask him where the motherfucking water main was. It was right where I thought it was after all. I had just been too tired or drunk to see it.

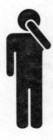 I zombie-shuffled to the bathroom to clean myself up, but there was no toilet paper. I went to get in the shower, but the water was still shut off.

Korma Karma

ASH J.

For my thirtieth birthday I'd invited a bunch of friends to
my local pub. My girlfriend and I were the first to arrive and
I took the opportunity to go to the loo. To be honest – and
I couldn't admit this to my girlfriend – I'd been feeling a bit
grim all day since heroically eating an entire Scotch bonnet
chilli during a romantic curry dinner the previous evening.
(Blokes might recognize the scenario. I'd said, 'I bet you I
can eat this whole chilli.' She said, 'I don't really mind. I don't
think you should.' I stuck the whole thing in my mouth while
she rolled her eyes and went back to her korma.)

Anyway, it seemed that now was the moment for my
comeuppance. I'd just got into the gents when my mate
George came in, having just arrived at the pub, and after a
hello and all that he headed for the only cubicle. Obviously
I couldn't stand there patiently waiting for him to have a shit
– unwritten rule – so I had to pretend I was just in there for
a wee.

But I'd only been at the urinal for a couple of seconds when
I began to be troubled by a feeling of impeding colonic
doom. Ignoring all the rules, written or otherwise, I yelled

at George to get out of the cubicle. He told me to fuck off – whereupon I entirely lost control sphinctorially. Shit ran all down my jeans and all over my socks and shoes. Of course this is when George finally re-emerged, laughing at first but then going wide-eyed with horror and disgust. I pushed past him – not easy in my state – and told him to go out to my girlfriend and cover for me. I cleaned myself up as best I could with scrappy bits of bog roll but there was just no fixing this mess.

I snuck out of the pub through a side door, where by now a bunch of my mates were gathered having a fag, and they watched as I scuttled away at speed. There was no way I was going to be allowed on a bus looking and smelling as I did, so I walked the half-hour back to my house under cover of darkness. I took off my trousers, socks and shoes in my front garden and chucked them in a wheelie bin, then showered and went immediately to bed.

I am told my thirtieth birthday party was a right laugh.

SOS

<u>DAVE P.</u>

I was taking a shit one time and the turd was so long and hard that it hit the bottom of the toilet before it had lost contact with my body. I had essentially created a solid shit column that had nowhere to go. Sure enough, and as anyone familiar with the fate of the *Titanic* will appreciate, the log cracked under the pressure and fell forwards, depositing itself onto the back of my scrotum. For a few stunned seconds I just sat there with a girthy turd leaning against the back of my balls, and then had to stand up to allow the thing to complete its tragic demise.

That was an interesting clean-up job.

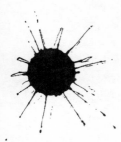

House of Horror

PAUL G.

My friend Stuart thought he'd hit the jackpot when he moved into a house share with four girls, but alas he hadn't reckoned with the daily loo lottery that came as part of the deal. He soon worked out a system for getting equal visitation rights to the bathroom, amid all the hair washing and horoscope reading the girls liked to do in there, but one chilly Monday morning he overslept and missed his slot.

Things were beginning to feel a little urgent in his bowels but there was no question of going outside (it was January) or running to the nearest pub (it was 7 a.m.), so he hatched the only plan he could come up with in his increasingly frenzied state: he would go down to the basement and shit into a plastic bag.

Bag in hand, he ran down there and hid behind the stairs. But the instant relief he felt at finally being able to let it all out was brutally cut short, mid-squeeze, when another of the female housemates descended into the basement to do her laundry. There was nothing to do but remain in a crouching position with arse and various other things dangling and hope to escape detection hidden under the stairs.

His housemate sorted her clothing neatly into colours and whites, then loaded the machine. Then she turned to take previously laundered clothing out of the dryer and folded it nicely into various piles, then closed the dryer door and tidied away all the detergent before finally fucking off upstairs. All the while Stu was crouched in increasing agony, peering through the steps and trying not to rustle the poo-filled bag.

As soon as his housemate returned upstairs he finished what he had started a number of minutes previously, wiped using an old rag and stretched his cramped legs. He tied the bag, opened the back door at the top of the basement steps and launched the evidence over the fence into the neighbour's back yard.

All well and good except that I was said neighbour. The reason he was telling me this story is because I found a bag full of human shit exploded on my patio.

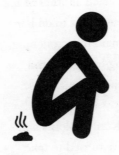

Sprung

OLLIE

It was the first sunny morning of spring and in my exuberance I'd decided to skip the bus and instead walk the half-hour to work. About ten minutes in, I remembered why I never did this: if I'd taken the bus I'd have been at the office enjoying my post-coffee morning bowel evacuation by now. As it was, I was all caffeined up with nowhere to go.

I told myself I could make it but my guts insisted otherwise. But what could I do? I was on a suburban street in a business suit, with parents and kids scootering their way to school all around me.

Suddenly I saw my opportunity. I'm ashamed to say I dashed into the narrow pathway between two houses, pulled down my trousers and did my extracurricular business right there. I had to rip one of the arms off my shirt to use as toilet paper.

In the middle of all this, as I was hovering bare-arsed and rending my garments, a little old lady popped her head out of the side door of one of the houses. She was carrying a big bag of rubbish and I was creating something of an obstacle – quite a steaming pile of an obstacle, in fact.

'Hey!' she yelled. 'WHAT ARE YOU DOING?'

'SHITTING!' I yelled back, figuring honesty was the best policy in the circumstances. She had eyes, after all.

'You're an animal!' she screamed. 'An animal! AN ANIMAL! ANIMAAAAAL!' – and so on, at ever greater volume until I could pull myself together and run away.

The guys in my office didn't believe a word of it until I took off my jacket to reveal my ruined shirt.

I blame the parents

SARAH F.

Let's clarify one thing before I commence: I do not poo at work. I've never been able to get over the public nature of it, and went through eight years of working life without this ever causing considerable issues. That lasted until this year.

My baby daughter stays at her child minder's home during the week while I'm at work and I collect her on my way home each day. Already as I left the office, I had rumblings of needing to go to the loo, but this is nothing out of the ordinary for someone who holds it in all day at her desk. By the time I got off the bus at the other end, however, I already felt the situation escalating to something awful. It is a fifteen-minute walk from the bus stop to the child minder's house, and another fifteen minutes from there to my home. I broke out into a shuffling jog.

The further I waddled, the worse the situation became. I knew there was no way of making the walk home any faster, and yet I also knew that my body could not possibly clench for another thirty agonizing minutes. I began to sweat.

In useless desperation, I called my husband's mobile while he was at work.

'Can you come and collect me? I'm really about to shit myself,' I sobbed down the phone. He was both incredulous and in a meeting.

The panic rose and I power-marched on until I reached the child minder's house, by this point the blotchy eyes of a madwoman complementing well my general erratic demeanour. The only thing worse than pooing at work is doing so in someone else's house so, despite my desperate situation, I couldn't bring myself to sully her bathroom. I barely made eye contact, grabbed my baby without even putting a coat on her – it was January – and left in a matter of seconds.

As I continued, the endless stretch of residential roads spread out before me, it seemed like I was never getting nearer to my home, no matter how much further I walked. Something terrible and immediate was about to occur.

Now it just so happens that on this day I was wearing tights, over which I had a very short women's romper suit and a long, dark trench coat. I looked down at my baby in her pram in front of me, and considered that any ghastly smell could easily be blamed on her for the remaining ten minutes of my walk home. Then I considered my outfit: the short romper suit was not ideal, but the tights and the long coat were certainly the perfect sartorial choice for a professional woman wishing to discreetly shit herself in the street.

Which is what I did.

Just a little bit – but just enough to abate any immediate (further) disaster. As I wandered happily down the road, I remember feeling so liberated after the short relief – so much so that as I paused at the traffic light crossing, I actually shat myself again out of choice. This was turning into something of a hobby.

When I finally reached home, I ran to the bathroom, sat my confused daughter down on the floor, as I threw everything into the shower and scrubbed like Lady Macbeth. When my husband got home later on to find me showered and all my clothes in the washing machine, he nervously asked how my journey home had gone.

'Oh, it was fine,' I said, and we've never spoken of it since.

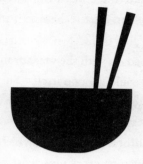

All-you-can-poo

RICHARD S.

When I was in my teens, my family went out for lunch in
China Town in London. Being an eager sixteen-year-old,
I filled my plate several times over from the all-you-can-eat
buffet as though I had never been fed before. We did some
touristy things in the afternoon and then made the journey
home in the car.

I started to feel a bit odd during the afternoon, but put it
down to having eaten my bodyweight in sweet and sour
chicken. It was as we got into the car that my stomach
started to gurgle unsettlingly. We had a forty-minute drive
ahead of us, and I thought I would ride it out – but every
bump and turn in the road made my bubbling belly jerk.

'Is there anywhere we can stop?' I asked my parents hopefully, and alerted them to my malaise.

We pressed on with the journey for a while, hoping that my body could contain itself – but I was not to be successful. As I contorted my body and crossed my legs in the back, I was sweating and panicking while my father scoured the street for a restaurant in which I might relieve myself. I was clenching every muscle in my body to control the rippling in my guts.

The car came to a screeching halt outside a small cafe, and I ran inside clutching my stomach. The sudden movement had parted my legs more than they had moved for the last half hour, and just as I blurted out, 'CAN I USE YOUR TOILET?' a loud splattering fart resounded around the empty cafe. I could feel that my legs were wet.

I saw the mouth of the solitary waitress drop as I waddle-ran towards the bathroom, each step forcing out further claps from my arse, with shit running down my legs and leaving an undeniable trail behind me. I fumbled the cubicle door lock, ripped down my trousers and sprayed shit all over the toilet, wall and floor with a long, satisfied groan. When the main disaster was over, I threw my ruined pants and socks into the cubicle bin, and made an ineffectual attempt to remedy the unusable bathroom.

Taking off my jumper to tie around my waist and hide my brown, wet trousers, I sheepishly emerged back into the cafe with blushing teenage apologies to the waitress and quietly sat back in the car.

'Everything alright, dear?' my mother asked.

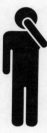 **The car came to a screeching halt outside a small cafe, and I ran inside clutching my stomach.**

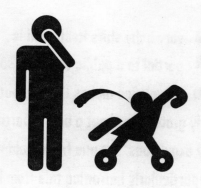

PART TEN:
AND ONE
ABOUT A
BABY . . . .

Every baby shits itself, and is partial to a public vom. And so its prevalence means there is nothing overly grotesque about a baby's particular daily expulsions. But one friend told me this particularly harrowing tale from last Christmas that deserves to be retold.

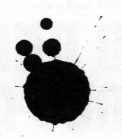

Baby, it's cold outside

SARAH

I had recently had my first child and didn't really have a clue what to do with him. To make matters worse we had just relocated to a village in northern Scotland and it was winter, which added an extra layer of farce to the already unbelievable amount of time it took me to achieve the smallest practical task.

Since Christmas was far from my mind, I had left my preparation until the last possible moment, and suddenly found myself home alone on the morning of 24 December with no turkey and some imminent in-laws. I rang round the local butchers, farmers and even supermarkets to no avail, and in my panic ended up placing an order for the last bird in some pop-up Christmas warehouse thirty miles away.

It took me hours to get there with the baby in tow and just as I triumphantly took my place in the deli queue of the chaotic tinsel-filled warehouse, with the child in my arms as I hadn't yet figured out how to work the expensive pram on my own, he chose his moment to execute one of those pootastrophes that makes new parents consider adoption. It was an explosion of hot shit all up his back and down his legs, gradually seeping out through the fabric of his clothes – and in through mine.

There was no way I was going to let this dirty protest scupper my chances of getting my hands on the turkey – my mother-in-law was arriving in two hours – so I stood firm in the queue with an angry and increasingly putrid child for the next twenty minutes. Then, carrying my two babies – one frozen, one dripping shit – I followed the signs to what I can only assume served as an abattoir washroom eleven months of the year, but which was now masquerading as the ladies' loo. It was all steel surfaces and bracing draughts and the child screamed bloody murder as I popped him down next to tomorrow's lunch and whipped all his clothes off. Needless to say, he peed in my face.

It was an explosion of hot shit all up his back and down his legs, gradually seeping out through the fabric of his clothes.

We had barely re-emerged into the shop when the half-hour of frantic crying took its inevitable toll and my son spray-puked warm milk all down my back and over a display table of festive handicrafts fashioned by local children, one of whom was in the middle of showing Grandma her painted-egg Santa.

Having ruined Christmas for a number of people, not least myself, I legged it out to the car with my prize turkey and, sadly, my stinking, unapologetic baby. It truly is a Christmas miracle that he's still with us today.

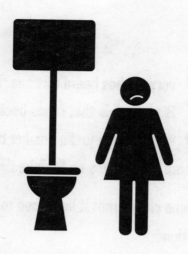

PART ELEVEN:
THE CLASSIC

Everyone has heard this one. The story is so terrible that it has become a thing of folklore in just a number of years, and there are even videos on YouTube depicting it.

Everyone claims that it happened to a friend of a friend.

Well I'm not going to claim that — because it actually happened to a friend of a friend's friend, who I have promised to keep anonymous in return for her first-hand account of the world's worst date ...

ANONYMOUS

(IT STARTS WITH O.)

This happened bloody years ago. I was on a first date with
a guy and all seemed to be going splendidly. We went to
a bar for a bottle of wine, followed by unplanned cocktails
and I ended up spending the night at his place.

The following morning, I woke up feeling several shades of
awful, and found him getting ready to leave. He explained he
had to go to work, but that I was more than welcome to stay
in bed a bit longer and to push the door locked when I left.

He clearly trusted me, and I was too hungover to move,
so I stayed put. When I eventually got up, I went to the
bathroom to sort myself out before starting the journey
home. And figuring he wouldn't be back for hours, I decided
that I could get away with doing a post-hangover poo here.

Except this one wouldn't go away. The bloody thing wouldn't
flush. I couldn't bear the idea of him coming home to find
it in his toilet, so decisive action needed to be taken. I'm not
quite sure what I was thinking, but the panic had set it.

I took a plastic bag from the kitchen, wrapped it round my hand inside out, and just grabbed the thing from the toilet bowl and tied it up inside the bag, so I could dispose of it anywhere outside.

I finished getting ready, and gathered my things, including the offensive bag. I left him a note on the kitchen table about how tremendous the night had been and left him my mobile number.

I left the flat, slammed the door shut as instructed, and then froze.

My left hand was empty. I knew instantly that I had left the wet bag of turd sitting next to my note on the kitchen table.

I took a plastic bag from the kitchen, wrapped it round my hand inside out, and just grabbed the thing from the toilet bowl.

Also by Michael O'Mara Books:

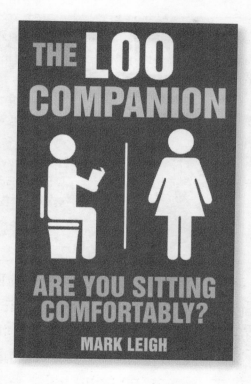

The Loo Companion
Mark Leigh
ISBN: 978-1-84317-631-2 in paperback print format
ISBN: 978-1-84317-817-0 in ePub format
ISBN: 978-1-84317-818-7 in Mobipocket format
£7.99

Also by Michael O'Mara Books:

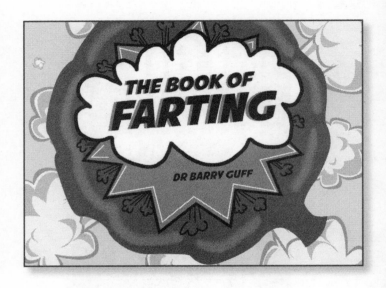

The Book of Farting
Dr Barry Guff
ISBN: 978-1-78243-180-0
£4.99